MEMOIRS OF A GYM RAT

One man's 20-year journey through the bowels of the health club industry.

Max Hawthorne

For Maria C., Connie T., and Nancy H. – the tiger lilies of my youth.
Here's to torn tongues, fear of "the big guy," and catsuits.
And what might have been.

"Truth is like the town whore. Everybody knows her, but nonetheless, it's embarrassing to meet her on the street."

-Wolfgang Borchert, The Outsider

CONTENTS

INTRODUCTION

The word was *vagina*.

I was sitting in my office at the health club doing the usual (admiring shapely females, texting family and friends, blabbing on the phone, etc.) when the door swung open and a gorgeous blonde suddenly burst in.

For our purposes, we'll call her "Ellen."

Ellen was a tiny little thing, only a smidgen over five feet. But her expensive sunglasses, five inch heels, and breasts the size of ripe cantaloupes, made a big impression. I gave her my full and immediate attention.

"Good afternoon," I said.

To my disappointment, Ellen remained in my doorway with her stiletto-clad feet spread wide apart, one hand on her hip. She looked about my tiny office and made a show of sniffing the air, like a bloodhound tracking its quarry.

"It smells pretty in here," she said. Before I could tell her that it was one of those plug-in air fresheners, she added, "It smells like *vagina*. Max, have you had _vagina_ in your office today?"

Momentarily taken aback, I managed only a hesitant "No . . ." But then I rebounded, adding, "At least, none of any quality." I fixed her with an intense stare and a shit-eating grin. "That is . . . not until *now*."

Ellen nodded. "Exactly." Beaming like a cat about to swallow a canary, she let my door swing silently closed. Then, without another word, she plopped herself down in the chair across from me and crossed her legs.

And thus began a typical day at work for me . . .

WHY FITNESS?

It's a question I've been asked many times. Given my family's long established predisposition for becoming doctors and lawyers, how the hell did I end up working in the fitness industry?

The answer is simple; like many people, I'd grown up with only one career in mind – and it didn't work out.

My childhood dream had been to be a veterinarian, a goal I nearly achieved. I worked part-time as a prominent vet's assistant, learning the business and assisting in surgeries, while maintaining a 3.9 GPA.

Unfortunately, I discovered that being a veterinarian wasn't everything I'd imagined. It wasn't about giving kittens vitamins and putting Band-Aids on puppy paws. It was dirty, primitive work, with animals constantly dying on the operating table. I also learned that vets earned much of their income by "disposing" of unwanted pets via lethal injection. These animals do not want to die, and will fight you tooth and claw to stay alive.

In the end, I couldn't stomach coming home covered in blood and hair, with the screams of dying dogs and cats echoing in my ears.

I quit my job at the vet's and dropped out of college. I started bumming around and working odd jobs. Eventually, my empty wallet and money-hungry landlord joined forces to remind me that I needed a steady paycheck. After some soul searching, I decided to turn something I enjoyed into a career – working in physical fitness.

What could be more logical? I lived for working out, so making it my job would be a pleasure rather than a chore. I'd already been exercising for eight years, and it would give me the chance to share my knowledge with others. I'd motivate my clients by showing them how I started off as a skinny, malnourished teen weighing only 130 lbs. (at 6'1") and transformed myself into a 195 pound athlete. Becoming a personal trainer, and helping other people, seemed like a sensible, even noble, thing to do.

With that in mind – and knowing absolutely nothing about the well-lubricated meat grinder that awaited me – I eagerly applied to one of the local chains.

And thus it began . . .

QUALIFICATIONS/INDUSTRY OVERVIEW

*B*y writing this book, I want to provide potential/current/former health club members with a no-holds-barred, behind-the-scenes look at the fitness industry, based on my own experiences. The numbers of people currently attending health clubs are staggering. As of the date this was written, there are over 26,000 health clubs in the U.S. alone, with more than 50 million members.

I was employed in the fitness field for twenty years, in a variety of locations. Over the course of my decades-long career I worked in eight different health clubs, ranging from 13,000 to 40,000 square feet. For the purposes of this book we'll call them Empirical Sports Clubs ("Empirical Sports"), Dinar Fitness, U.S. Amazing Fitness, and Caveat Sports Clubs ("Caveat Sports"). The largest fitness chains in the country owned six of them, while the remaining two were private labels.

Like most people starting out new to a field, I had to start at the bottom and work my way up from there. I certainly paid my dues.

Over the years, I wore many hats, from beleaguered floor instructor to sadistic personal trainer, all the way to General Manager. I ran facilities that hosted more than 10,000 members and learned all sorts of unpleasant corporate secrets along the way. I also discovered the disturbing things that went on in my clubs – things I wouldn't have believed possible, but which often happened right under clients' noses.

When I eventually realized that the only way to make money in fitness was via selling gym memberships, I changed gears. I busted my ass until I became one of the top salespeople in the industry, and also one of the most popular. Over a period of seventeen years I enrolled over 25,000 clients. While doing so I encountered some of the most interesting, attractive, bizarre, and depraved (if not outright insane) people I've ever met in my life.

Working in fitness changes people, and not just on the outside. When I first started in the industry, I was an innocent. I had naïve, preconceived notions about how health clubs operated; I believed they existed purely to benefit their clients with the gift of health. I quickly learned otherwise.

In fact, I ended up knowing too much.

In the pages of *Memoirs of a Gym Rat,* you will discover that many of the "crimes" I expose I'm guilty of committing myself. It's the truth, and I won't bother denying it. That's why I know all about the bad things that happen in gyms – because I did them. Why? It would be easy to explain myself by saying, "Peer pressure," "It's the nature of the beast," or "I'm a guy, what do you expect?" and leave it at that. But those would be cop-outs.

The truth is I was young and single, working in an industry filled with temptations. And I succumbed to them. I was a flawed person to begin with, but the job brought these weaknesses and imperfections to the fore. I did some mean, unethical things – and I grew to enjoy them. My personality changed, but not for the better. After a few years, I could barely recognize myself. When I look back at the person that I was it's like I'm looking back at a stranger. I thank God that the "man" I was then is not the man I am today.

Still, the following are truthful accounts of what I saw and did. You are about to discover what went on daily (sometimes behind closed doors, sometimes not) in the high-profile gyms where I worked. And, you will get an idea of what may be going on where *you* exercise. Although told with a warped sense of humor, much of the content of this book is shocking and not for the faint of heart. There is foul and explicit language, sexual innuendo, and situations that are frankly disgusting. Reader discretion is advised.

For those who do choose to peruse these pages, I hope *Memoirs of a Gym Rat* serves as a useful survival guide for any of you using a health club, working in the field, or considering doing so.

If not, maybe you'll have a few laughs.

Healthfully Yours,
Max Hawthorne

CHAPTER 1:

WORKING IN THE INDUSTRY

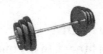

My first job in fitness was as a lowly floor instructor, working for a company called "Caveat Sports Clubs" in Brooklyn, New York.

The job itself almost didn't happen. I'd sent out lots of applications, but everyone kept giving me the runaround. Despite my years of bodybuilding and martial arts experience – and an enviable physique to boot – no one would give me the time of day. I continued to drop off resumes, but my follow-up calls remained unanswered. And when I did get a manager on the phone, they always said they were busy or refused to grant me an interview.

In the end, I was hired by accident. I was so frustrated that I finally went over the managers' heads. I called a new "super-club" in the area and asked to speak to the area manager. I was told his name was "Johnson," and, luckily enough, he was in and available.

When I got Johnson on the phone, I spouted about my dedication to fitness and years of experience. I told him I could work for him as a trainer, and would be the best there was, but unfortunately none of his people would give me a shot. I explained that, although we'd spoken previously, the manager at the nearby Brooklyn location wouldn't even interview me.

This was where fate stepped in – a fateful failure to communicate.

It turns out Johnson had a considerable ego. And when I said that *we'd* spoken previously, he assumed I meant that *he* and *I* had talked. In his faulty memory, he had wanted to hire me, sight unseen, but his subordinate hadn't granted the requisite interview.

Johnson grew genuinely angry at his manager for "defying" him. He told me to call the club and speak with the guy directly, per *his* instructions. I was to tell him I'd been sent by Johnson personally for a training position – and to get the ball rolling ASAP.

I did as he instructed. Obviously afraid of his boss, the manager hired me on the spot. When I arrived there was no interview at all. I just had to fill out an employee packet and they processed my paperwork while I waited.

I might have been accidentally hired, but I wasn't about to complain. I had the job I wanted, in a field I was dying to work in, and I was fired up. I was going to be the best trainer in the business and nothing would stand in my way.

STARTING AT THE "BOTTOM"

I was ecstatic to be working in fitness. In my mind I'd created a glittering version of what working in a health club would be like. All my preconceptions would quickly vanish.

On the train ride there, my mind soared. I imagined all the state-of-the-art equipment, the aerobics classes, and all those fit bodies moving in unison. I would be breathing air that was literally infused with health and vitality. I was totally pumped as I walked through the door.

Five minutes later, my General Manager introduced me to the club's floor manager, "Agatha," who I'd be answering to. She was a lean, hungry-looking aerobics instructor in her late thirties, with a flat stomach and an even flatter disposition.

Agatha gave me my first taste of what working in a gym was actually like. She looked me up and down like a piece of meat and ordered me to slowly spin around. After appraising me with a cool stare, she drew uncomfortably close. While I froze in fear, she ran her nails across my pectorals (deliberately grazing one nipple), and then gave my biceps an exploratory grope. God knows what she would have done if her boss hadn't interrupted her. "Are you going to check his teeth, too?" he asked.

Apparently that only happens with horses.

Although I was shaken at being pawed over like some prize stud bull, I soon discovered many more unexpected negatives that came with my new position. At the end of my shift I spent a good hour scrubbing off the coagulated grease and body hair from all the exercise equipment – gunk accumulated from sweaty gym patrons who failed to wipe down their machines after use.

Far worse was the salary: $5.50 an hour. Even after putting in full work weeks, I couldn't make enough money to cover my expenses. Rent, train fare, utilities . . . everything added up, and week after week I found myself falling deeper into the hole. It's a bad look to come home with your girl-friend and discover that your electricity has been turned off.

Being a floor instructor had an even bigger downside: the company barred me from doing personal training – the reason I took the job in the first place. The only exception to this was the "group orientations" they were required by law to give new members (a one-time brief in-troduction to a series of eight antiquated weight machines). Before I could find clients and start doing real PT sessions, I had to get my certi-fication. That meant spending three months scrubbing down machines before I'd be certified through Caveat Sports' in-house program. This sucked, especially since I was better informed than 90% of their "certi-fied" instructors.

Still, I had to pay my dues, so I spent my days wearing a forced smile. Despite the fact that I wasn't technically allowed to train people, I ended up taking the most bewildered gym members under my wing and helping them out. And believe me, they were happy to have me. At first there was just one or two, but soon their numbers grew. Eventually, I was training doz-ens of enthusiastic clients for free. It was a boon to me as well; it solved my biggest problem – how to look busy.

I quickly discovered the vital importance of "looking busy." My job de-pended on it. Believe me, no one will pay you even $5.50 an hour to scratch yourself – no matter how good looking you are or where it itches. And Agatha, for whatever reason, loved sneaking up on the gym floor to catch me goofing off. She was always looking to write someone up. Maybe it was how she justified her job. I honestly don't know.

Regardless, I became a master of putting on appearances, even when I had absolutely nothing to do. I could point out every security mirror in the place; I developed radar, sonar, and eyes in the back of my head. Even if nobody needed help, I could always "be on my way to report" a faulty weight machine that was a potential lawsuit waiting to happen.

I learned something else from working in fitness: Never turn your back on anyone, because that's where the knife goes.

KEEPER OF THE HOUSE

As I settled into my position as an instructor, I got to know my various co-workers. I tried to learn as much as I could about them and their jobs. Besides being polite, it made sense – I wanted to know everything there was to know about my new field.

I soon discovered a rather poorly kept secret: housekeepers are the backbone of any fitness facility. They're the ones that keep the place looking good and running. They keep the floors free of dust bunnies and coyotes (you know – the really big ones that *eat* the dust bunnies), the mirrors shiny, and the toilets and showers sterile.

Unfortunately, like floor trainers, they are the least well paid. It's ironic that those that do the hardest work get the least compensation. As a result, the people that end up being hired to keep the place clean are usually not of the highest caliber.

It's a mathematical certainty: minimum wage = minimal effort.

To make matters worse, besides hiring whoever they can find, many gyms make a second mistake. They skimp on hours for housekeeping, leaving the place short-staffed or even unattended. Why? I have absolutely no idea. Maybe they think the overflowing toilets in the locker room are going to magically unclog themselves.

Author's Note: Clogged toilets are <u>*nothing*</u>*. As you'll discover, I've seen things while touring club locker rooms that made me run screaming.*

The first housekeeper I met at Caveat Sports worked full-time in the men's locker room. He was quite the malingerer. I used to call him "Roamer," because that's what he did all day – roam around the place, instead of doing his job. I constantly caught him hiding in closets, sneaking sandwiches, and taking naps in bathroom stalls.

One fine day, a client's child decided to take a dump in one of our sales reps offices. Roamer was called to action. When he came upstairs and saw this little girl's turd staring up at him he shrugged and started walking away. The sales associate, understandably shaken, tried to keep her cool. She calmly asked Roamer to do his job. He rubbed his fingers together, and the meaning was clear: "Give me money." After a heated argument (including a threat to report him to the manager) he finally did what he was paid to do, but he was hardly enthusiastic about it.

A year later, I had a similar incident with Roamer inside the men's locker room. To my horror, I discovered that someone had relieved themselves inside one of the shower stalls (this type of thing happens a lot in gyms). When I saw the mess and pointed it out to Roamer, figuring he'd take care of it, he tried the same shake-down routine with me.

At this point, I'd moved up in the world. I was the Assistant Manager of the facility, so I had authority over the little shit (pun intended). It was just the two of us in the locker room, and I wasn't in the mood. I'm not naturally violent, but I'd put up with his insubordination for far too long. I moved close to him and whispered in his ear that if he *didn't* do his job I wouldn't report him; I would beat the snot out of him, then and there. And I meant it.

During my years at Caveat Sports I had many interesting experiences involving Roamer, but my all-time favorite took place a few months later. I was seated in a sales office, jawing with one of my colleagues, when he came in to complain about a fellow housekeeper.

You have to understand that Roamer was an unkempt, scruffy-looking guy. He smelled like a mixture of bad body odor and bug spray, his face was usually dirty, and his "white" pants were a light shade of gray from all the ground-in grease and crud.

My co-worker and I sat there, breathing through our mouths as we politely listened to Roamer's complaints. Then, before my disbelieving eyes, a cockroach crawled out from the bottom cuff of Roamer's pants, made its way up his leg, and disappeared into his hip pocket.

And he was oblivious to it.

I was horrified, and half-hoping I'd imagined it. But once Roamer left the office my co-worker turned to me, her eyes huge. "Holy shit! Did you *see* that?"

"See what?" I replied, not willing to volunteer anything.

"That roach!" she exclaimed. "Did you see that big cockroach run up his pants leg and go in his pocket?"

"You saw it too?"

"Yes," she said, obviously relieved she was as sane (or insane) as me. "I can't believe it. There's a grown man walking around with a live roach chilling out in his pocket."

"Maybe it's a pet," I volunteered.

I tried to shake the visual out of my head. But I just couldn't stop myself from thinking about what would happen when Roamer went to McDonald's for his usual lunch. I pictured him reaching into his pocket for money, only to find his six-legged friend seated hungrily on top of his wad.

THE HUMMINGBIRD

As you might know, many health clubs offer massage therapy as a paid option for members. It lets them pamper their clients while increasing ancillary (non-dues generated) revenue. The first massage therapist I met was also back when I was a floor instructor at Caveat Sports. His name was "Dmitry," but I refer to him as the "Hummingbird." I ran into him one day as he was coming out of the sauna. He was buck naked and soaked with sweat.

Now, I usually don't check out other men's privates, but in this case I couldn't help myself. I've been in and out of men's locker rooms for decades, I've seen a fair share of porn, but Dmitry had the tiniest penis I've ever seen. All he had was a tiny, mushroom-like head – like a button glued to his lower abdomen – and that was it.

I blinked a few times and kept on walking. I tried to forget, but the Hummingbird continued to haunt me. He'd just come out of the sauna, so there was no possibility of any "shrinkage." I couldn't understand how the guy could urinate, let alone copulate. How could he ever reproduce? After all, you can't score a home run if you don't round first.

The Hummingbird ended up hating my guts (no, it's *not* because I told everyone he was hung like a hamster – although I probably did). He used to use the club's overhead mike system to drum up customers for his massage business. You'd hear announcements like: *"Attention, male members. If you want beautiful, relaxing massage come to men's locker room, ask for Dmitry."*

My manager at the time, "Robert," was a bit of a clown. He was obsessed with impersonations and used this talent to make fun of people. Robert could precisely replicate the Hummingbird's voice, Russian accent and all.

Whenever Dmitry was out of the club, Robert would hop on the loudspeaker and do *his* version of our massage therapists' announcement. *"Attention, male members. If you want beautiful, relaxing hand job – um . . . I mean,* massage *– come to men's locker room. Ask for Dmitry."*

The guffaws ended, however, when the Hummingbird came back early from break one day and heard one of the announcements. When confronted, my cowardly manager not only denied any responsibility; he had the balls to tell our infuriated masseuse that *I* was the one doing it.

Editor's Note: There are few things in life more awkward than an angry naked man with a tiny penis trying to pick a fight with you over something you didn't do.

POWER CORRUPTS

During my first few months at Caveat Sports I learned a lot about the people I worked with. I realized they weren't the dedicated, hard-core fitness professionals I expected them to be. Most of them had no background in the field and had taken their jobs purely out of need or convenience. Moreover, they spent most of their time making fun of clients behind their backs, or gossiping about each other's sex lives.

The staff suffered from a general lack of moral character, as well as a pattern of blatant sexual behavior that, although concealed in the beginning, soon became embarrassingly obvious.

And it went all the way to the top.

My manager Robert was guilty of an astonishing array of sexual practices that took place right in the club. Besides running the gym, he also worked in a few area bars and nightclubs. Since he had the keys to our club, and since he didn't want to get caught cheating on his fiancé (or just didn't want to spend money on motels), he used to bring intoxicated girls back to the gym in the middle of the night for hardcore, one-on-one "workouts."

Although I didn't know who the perpetrator was, I knew that *something* was going on. One morning, I even found used condoms strewn in the Jacuzzi and around the pool. Obviously, the nasty things got there somehow. I reported my discovery to housekeeping, who told Robert. While passing his office later, I overheard him bragging to someone on the phone about how he'd forgotten to clean up after his latest middle-of-the-night conquest. He seemed to find my discomfort very amusing.

Needless to say, I wasn't going anywhere near the hot tub after that . . .

UNEXPECTED PERKS

Although being a floor instructor at Caveat Sports was difficult and demeaning work, I soon discovered I had access to the most amazing job perk imaginable:

Limitless sex.

Yes, you read that right. Based on the things I've seen over the years, I've come to the inescapable conclusion that sex is the reason most people join a health club in the first place.

A few weeks into my job, I was constantly hit on by the health club's female population. At first, I thought it was my ego talking – or I was losing my mind. I couldn't believe that so many women were interested in me, especially these ones. They were all fit and shapely; if I bumped into any of them in a dance club, I wouldn't have expected her to give me the time of day. Yet in the gym, I got plenty of attention

I began to reciprocate. The women there were *definitely* not shy. I guess to them I was something different: tall and personable, with a winning smile and a singular wit (I was modest, too). Also, as I wasn't from New York, I didn't have that traditional Brooklyn accent. But having had only a handful of relationships, I was naïve when it came to members of the opposite sex. Especially these surprisingly aggressive female gym rats, who had the exact same thing on their minds as the juiced-up males of their species (and there's *nothing* wrong with that).

I finally agreed to go out with this tall, well-built blonde girl. Her idea of a date consisted of inviting herself to my apartment to "watch TV." The moment she discovered I lived alone, she picked me up and threw me eight feet onto the bed, then pounced on me and started ripping my clothes off. I was astonished by her strength. Panic set in! For a few seconds, I resisted. Then I stopped and thought: *why the _hell_ am I struggling?*

The girl was surprisingly laid back about the whole thing. She told me that she would like us to keep hooking up, but that it should be a casual thing. She thought we should both see other people; in fact, she insisted on it. If I was fine with that, she was game to continue.

I was stunned, yet intrigued. The manager of my old gym at college had once told me how one of his sales guys was sleeping with five different women at the same time. I remembered the guy. He was animated and amusing, but he wasn't exactly an Adonis. I thought to myself, could this be possible?

And if *he* could pull it off, why couldn't I?

Without further ado, I threw myself into the fray. I got one girl's phone number after another's. It was like diving into a mountain of cocaine; I was quickly addicted. After a few weeks I was juggling six attractive women and sleeping with all of them. It was absolutely amazing. I realized that my facility was absolutely *swarming* with available hotties. It was like the place had ass on tap. For the first time in my life, I was drowning in babes, and the delicious deluge more than made up for my paltry salary. Whereas other men my age focused on their careers and making money, my primary goal was getting laid by as many women as possible – and the hotter the better.

In retrospect, I had turned into a total sexual addict, but what did I know?

My being broke didn't make a difference. Those magnificent she-cats weren't interested in being wined and dined; they couldn't care less about such things. It was obvious. Whenever I asked a girl what she wanted to do, I'd get the same, silkily purred response. *"Whatever you want is fine, baby."* Which translates to: *"I want to go back to your place and ride you until your toes curl."*

There had to be *some* illusion of an actual first date, so I would do the gentlemanly thing and suggest we get a video and some take-out and chill at my place. Of course, the Chinese food never got ordered, and only the first five minutes of any given movie ever got watched, but what the heck – two dollars was a cheap price to pay for great sex.

There was a downside to juggling so many women: it affected me psychologically. It became impossible for me to get attached to someone. My emotions were so divided up that I felt nothing for the person I was with. Plus, I had to keep track of all the lies I was telling, and to whom.

I kept a "cheat sheet" in my wallet with the names and numbers of all the women I was seeing. I *had* to; it was the only way I could keep track. I put little checks next to their names to make sure I'd called them, and jotted down notes, excuses and alibis for upcoming dates.

The biggest problem, however, was the ego factor. As the notches on my bedpost grew, so did my head; I became an obnoxious, swelled-up egomaniac. And I had such an unlimited supply of women that I took them all for granted. I didn't treat them well, and if a girl got on my nerves, I simply crossed her off my list. I called it "culling the herd."

Things really got out of hand. One morning, after sending my thoroughly pleased date on her way, it occurred to me that I'd slept with three women in one day. Still in my pajamas, I raised my fists overhead, Rocky-style, and pranced around in front of my apartment like I'd just won the heavyweight crown.

Needless to say, I'd become something unpleasant.

In my own defense, I never meant anyone harm. I thought all the girls I dated were awesome – at least before the falling out. I was just a young guy with a lot of hormones and a personal harem. An unlimited buffet of love was spread out willingly before me. And I was *very* hungry.

TOO CLOSE FOR COMFORT

When the women you're dating frequent the place where you work, you're taking your life in your own hands. But I was young and stupid, so discretion was not a priority.

After a few close calls, I started to wise up and learned how to properly manage my paramours. "Sure, I'd love for you to stay over, but my dad's coming in the morning, and I don't want his first impression of you to be you walking around my apartment wearing my t-shirt," or "Listen, I really care about you, but I'm not allowed to date women from the gym. It's very important that we keep our relationship a secret. Otherwise I could lose my job, and then I'd never see you again."

Worked like a charm.

I also learned that regular gym members usually have set schedules and routines: they either come in the morning, lunchtime, or in the evening. So I started dating girls from different shifts. It reduced the chances of them seeing me with someone else or striking up a conversation with each other while doing cardio.

They called me all day long, sometimes two or three at a time. As my popularity grew, so did my hubris: Paula Abdul's *"Cold Hearted"* was my theme song. At one point, I was dating a sexy Italian receptionist ("Kristin"), a cute Filipino nursery attendant ("Anita"), and a hot Ukrainian aerobics instructor ("Tanya") on top of it. When Kristin started giving me a hard time about my cavalier attitude, I foolishly decided to teach her a lesson. Instead of breaking up with her, I handed her a pair of Anita's earrings and asked if she'd be kind enough to return them.

Kristin flipped out, and I upped the ante. I told her that I'd seen her, Anita and Tanya talking the day before – and that it warmed the cockles of my heart to see the three of them bonding like that. "You all have *so* much in common." Needless to say, the first "Max Haters Club" was formed shortly thereafter.

I learned a valuable lesson from this. Do *not* date the girls you work with – *especially* if you're stupid enough to open your mouth.

I had a far more dangerous close call a few weeks later. I was loitering in the free weight room, sneaking in a few sets of biceps curls. In mid-set, I got a phone call, then another, and another. Annoyed by the incessant interruptions, I headed for the exit, through a corridor that ran beside the aerobics room.

As I reached the doorway, I came to a screeching halt. Panic set in, followed by cold fear. Ahead and to the left were our three Stairmasters, lined side by side and facing the mirror. Three different girls, all of whom I was dating, were contentedly using the machines. I stared in disbelief. What were the odds?

I cursed and retreated back into the safety of the free weight room. There was no way out; I was trapped. They'd already spotted me and, worse, I now had calls coming in on *three* lines at once.

I rocked back on my heels as my mind did NASCAR-style laps. For a split-second, I considered walking out and facing the music. Fortunately, *that* suicidal notion vanished *real* quick. I've been shot at, I've fought off a hungry alligator, and I've forced my way out of a burning SUV seconds before it exploded (true stories), but nothing was like the fear I felt in that weight room. Those three chicks were stacked, packed and jacked. But I knew from personal experience that they also had tempers so foul only a complete fool would risk their wrath.

I'd never survive getting busted by *one* of them.

Finally, I hatched a plan borne of utter desperation. I waited for my next page, and then sprinted down the hall at top speed, my eyes deliberately focused straight ahead. I saw all three girls perk up in the mirror. I grinned madly and gave a random wave that could have been meant for anyone, then kept running.

As luck would have it, this combination of high speed and misdirection saved my profusely-sweating ass. Each of the girls assumed my wave was meant for her and her alone. Now the three Stairmaster neighbors had become potential rivals and I was safe, if just for the moment.

And so it went, day by day. It never occurred to me then that sex is like power; if not contained, the more you have, the worse you become. I just knew I was getting more ass than a toilet seat. Nothing fazed me. Not the fear of getting caught or even the emotional trauma I caused the girls who really liked me. After all, not every girl in the gym was just looking for a good time. Some of them actually cared.

DEADLIEST CATCH

Eventually, God taught me the error of my ways. I was dating this gorgeous Dominican girl. She was a thing of beauty, with breasts like grapefruits, eyes like emeralds, and a bootie most women would ritually sacrifice their best friend to have. We'll call her "Juliette." Besides some nice bath towels and amazing romps in the hay, Juliette gave me something else. Something far more personal.

Crabs!

Condoms don't protect you from the little monsters. Thinking it was only a bad case of jock itch, I ended up forwarding Juliette's little present to four other women. Then I had to call them all up and *confess*. And I don't want to even *touch* on the walk of shame to the counter of my amused local pharmacist.

Fortunately, I bounced back. My sunken spirits were buoyed by something looming on the horizon – something that I knew would free me from the hell of cleaning grimy weight machines and give me more money (and sex) to boot. I was moving up in the world, transcending to something far more prestigious. I was about to become that most dreaded and misunderstood of gym creatures . . .

A certified personal trainer.

SURVIVAL TIP #1:

This one's for the girls. Not to pigeonhole people, but it's fair to point out that most men working in gyms are pigs. Yes, that's right – pigs, pure and simple. Believe me, I know. As charming and personable as I was, I was one of the worst oinkers out there, and just about every guy I've ever worked with turned out to be almost as bad. Married or single, it didn't make a difference.

So keep that in mind, if you're dating or considering some-one who works in a health club. Odds are he (or she, for that matter) has slept with half the place already. If you're okay with being just another notch on someone's well-worn weight belt, then that's fine. All I ask is that you do yourself one, small favor. Use protection.

But remember, you can still catch crabs!

CHAPTER 2:

MY STINT AS A PERSONAL TRAINER

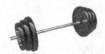

After attending a forty-hour class provided (for a fee) by Caveat Sports, I successfully passed my personal training certification course. I did well; in fact, I had the top score in the class.

I returned to my club and promptly got to work. Finally I could do some good for my clients; this was the reason I took the floor instructor job in the first place. As a bonus, I had the chance to earn a lot more money and wouldn't have to scrub down dirty machines (a nice perk).

I instantly signed up a half-dozen of the clients I'd been training for free; fortunately, they were eager to shell out money to work with me in a formal capacity. Word of my clients' success quickly spread. Within a month or two, I was booked solid for forty hours in advance.

Over the years, I've heard trainers at countless clubs complain they can't find clients or hit their "minimums" (quotas set by the club to pressure them into getting clients). I could never understand this. I never had a problem acquiring "fresh meat." All I had to do was wander around the gym floor until I found some poor slob doing an exercise so badly they were bound to hurt themselves. Then I stopped and helped them.

For the uninitiated, and based on my own experience, a lot of health clubs *deliberately* deny their clients personal training when they join, in order to herd them into paying for it. They usually give you an hour or two when you sign up, but that's it. Caveat Sports was even worse: one floor instructor would show large groups a half-hour-long "exercise routine." This was sufficient to shield them from being liable for client injuries. It also ensured that their clients were so clueless and desperate that, given the opportunity, they'd jump at paying for help.

I was astounded at how starved for knowledge most of my members were. Once they found out that not only could I show them how to do an exercise correctly, but that they could actually *feel* the benefits, they were *dying* to work with me.

All they needed to do was break out their checkbook.

SURVIVAL TIP #2

If you're joining a gym, make sure to find out how much help you'll get, especially if you're inexperienced and on a budget. Whereas most small businesses fail due to lack of capital, most workout routines fail because people don't know what they're doing. Gyms are mazes of equipment, weights and machines. New members become confused and overwhelmed, fail to make progress, and eventually get frustrated and quit (and usually still have to keep paying).

Most people need at least three hours of one-on-one instruction in order to learn a basic routine. Five would be better. Since most gyms pay their trainers floor hours only when they're not doing paid sessions, it wouldn't hurt to negotiate for some extra help when you're signing up. Tell your sales rep that you won't join unless you get some additional private training with your package. They may hem and haw, but the odds are they'll give you what you want in order to close the sale. Especially once you imply that you're afraid of injuring yourself . . .

Giving you PT won't cost them anything, and for you it may just mean the difference between success and failure.

IN-HOUSE HIJINKS

I quickly developed a reputation as the best trainer in the region. Success was great, but having so many back-to-back clients soon became problematic. I used to pray for cancelations so I could grab lunch or sneak in a workout.

Even though I was busy, scoring with girls stayed high on my list of priorities. It started to feel like a second job. My manager Robert was no stranger to womanizing; after all, he was the one leaving used prophylactics all over the place. It perplexed him, however, that I was so good at it.

Robert initiated a practical joke campaign against me. My overhead pages soon changed from "Attention staff: Max you have a phone call on line two," to "Attention staff: Max, your ego's on line two," or "Attention, Max's ego: lines two and three . . . Repeat, Max's ego, lines two and three."

Undaunted by these hijinks, I carefully prepared to retaliate. Robert had a crucial weakness: he loved to eat. But just as he was about to bite into a nice sandwich or slice of pizza, a potential client would invariably walk into Caveat Sports and ask about joining. Naturally, Robert couldn't sit there with a big plate of food in front of a potential commission, so he'd leave his meal on his desk and take his prospect into an adjacent office. Once he was in the middle of a sale, he wasn't going anywhere. I frequently came across his unguarded food. After a quick check to make sure the coast was clear, I'd pop in, take the biggest bite possible out of his virgin sandwich, and keep on cruising. It was a hungry trainer's version of a drive-by.

This went on for months, and it boggled my mind that Robert didn't realize what was going on. Finally, the day came where I made a move on his defenseless plate of KFC. Suddenly, a resounding "Stay away from my chicken!" reverberated from his office's speakerphone.

The jig was up.

WHAT A JOHNSON!

Over the years, I usually found that the biggest hypocrites in fitness are those in what is known as "supervisory positions." These are men and women who have been with a company for years and worked their way up the corporate ladder. Their titles might be Area Supervisor, Sales Manager, District Manager, or Area Manager (to name a few). They are usually responsible for six or eight facilities and answer to some sort of Regional Director or VP.

My first exposure to what supervisors are capable of was back when I was a floor instructor at Caveat Sports. As I mentioned earlier, I'd spoken to Johnson on the phone, back when I was trying to break into the business. I didn't know much about him at first, except that he ran a bunch of Brooklyn clubs.

As an instructor and trainer, I noticed that Johnson spent an inordinate amount of time at my facility. The first few times I saw him, I took note of the powerful effect he had on people. The moment he walked into our club, all of the staff instantly went on high alert. The manager alternated between scrambling to get things done and kissing Johnson's ass.

The rest of the employees, especially the salespeople, were in a state of panic. They stayed glued to the phones, cold-calling people left and right in an effort to appear hard at work.

Sometimes their maelstrom of calls would backfire. Johnson would settle into an office and sit there like a low-rent sultan, going over reports while receiving a generous massage from whichever well-built female staff member was available. When he reached for the phone and realized all the lines were taken, he'd go berserk.

I remember walking by and hearing him bellow, "Somebody hang up the fucking phone!"

I have to say, I was mighty glad I wasn't in sales back then.

As a trainer, I witnessed another incident involving Johnson – one that was way worse. Not only should he have been *fired* for what he did, but the victim could have sued as well. It was a weekend shift, a little after 9 a.m. I was cruising past the sales offices on my way to the aerobics studio. I saw Johnson swagger into the Assistant Manager's office. She was a really spiritual girl. I can't remember her name, but let's call her "Crystal."

I overheard Johnson ask Crystal how many sales she had on. "None," she nervously answered. Since her shift had only started fifteen minutes earlier, I didn't think that was a big deal. Obviously unhappy with her answer, however, Johnson started nosing around her office. Crystal tried to ignore him by staying glued to the phone and waking poor people up on a Saturday morning.

Suddenly, Johnson yanked open the top drawer of her filing cabinet and peered inside. An ugly expression crept across his face. "Look at this shit!" he snarled. "It's a fucking mess!"

Without another word, he ripped the whole filing cabinet drawer out and overturned it, dumping papers, files, pens, and paper clips – not to mention the entire contents of Crystal's purse – in a big pile all over the floor.

Ranting and raving, Johnson pulled out the remaining two drawers and upended them as well, leaving an enormous mess scattered throughout the office. Crystal fell on her knees, terrified and sobbing, while he stood over her with his arms folded across his chest and bellowed, "Now clean this shit up! And when you're finished, you're demoted and transferred downtown!"

Johnson's name should have been "Dick."

As a PT, I was fortunate enough not to work for Johnson, at least not directly. I still remember an encounter I had with him, back when I was a floor instructor. It was nearly closing time, and I was upstairs wiping down weight machines. He was working out, trying to pump up his less-than-intimidating physique. He knew about my reputation and asked if he could be a member of my "fan club." I fought down a smirk and politely offered to help him. I told him I'd be happy to build up that flat space where his chest was supposed to be -- free of charge.

From that point forward, there was little love lost between us. Our mutual dislike simmered until one day it exploded into open hostility, costing me my job, and him very nearly his teeth, but that takes place a few years (and chapters) later.

EXTREME TRAINING

There are two things I can unequivocally say about myself as a personal trainer. The first is that I was very good at it.

Over an eighteen month period, I transformed scores of people's bodies, improving their health and self-esteem in the process. I took one woman who was 40 lbs. overweight -- with the muscle tone of wet pasta -- and in six months turned her into a professional-caliber athlete. She was lean, mean, and as strong as half the guys in the gym.

At first, she scoffed at doing PT. That was, until she worked out on her own for six months and lost only a pound.

As luck would have it, her husband was so enamored with her new and improved physique that he promptly knocked her up. She regained all the weight I'd helped her shed.

You win some; you lose some.

The second thing I can say about myself is that, when it came to training my clients, I was a sadistic maniac. My staff nicknamed me "the Punisher," after the comic book antihero. I pushed people five times harder than they'd push themselves, and then some. Often I'd train two clients at a time (yes, double pay); while one of them did a set, the "resting" client ran a lap. Then they switched.

Talk about a rest interval!

CHARACTER SPOTLIGHT: LUCKY IN LOVE

One of my saddest PT-related stories happened while I was a trainer at Caveat Sports. I had a colleague who worked at a different location. I called him "Lucky."

He wasn't.

Lucky was a nice kid. He was young, athletic and good-looking, with chiseled features and big blue eyes, but he wasn't exactly the sharpest tool in the shed. He had an ongoing problem: his co-workers would wait for him to cash his paycheck, then sneak into his office and steal his money. The saddest part was that Lucky *knew* someone was doing it, yet he kept leaving his wallet where it could be ransacked.

As a result, the guy was constantly broke with rent to pay. Fortunately for him, he had a wealthy female client who was hopelessly in lust with him. She wanted that beach boy body of his more than anything. When she heard about the robbery, she *instantly* offered to give him the five hundred dollars he needed to avoid eviction. There was just one teeny, tiny condition.

Lucky had to sleep with her.

Now, for anyone who thinks this was a great opportunity, keep in mind Lucky was a twenty-year-old jock that girls went absolutely crazy over. He also had a beautiful girlfriend whom he was madly in love with, and the client in question bore a striking resemblance to a camel.

Sadly, poor Lucky was out of options. He was forced to give in to his client's desire and allow her to satiate her vile, pagan lusts with his nubile flesh. I felt bad for the guy. He told me he was so disgusted by the experience he vomited afterward. Even worse, his cash kept getting stolen, so he had to keep putting out for this woman. He never seemed to learn from his mistakes, or have the motivation to make sure it never happened again.

I always wondered if his lusty client was in on the scam and made sure he kept getting robbed just so she could keep her claws in him.

INTRUDER ALERT

When it comes to brutal workouts there is one incident I really relish. I was putting one of my regulars through a particularly hellish routine: doing strip-sets on the seated row machine.

Strip-sets entail starting off with a weight a client can do a certain number of reps with. When they've reached the point of failure, you immediately lower the weight (say from 100 to 80 pounds). Then, you make them do another set to failure without resting. Then you drop the weight again. And so forth. It makes them push way past normal thresholds and recruits tons of additional muscle fibers. Granted, it's not something you should do often, and it feels like a blowtorch running up and down your muscles, but used properly it works – and works well.

My client "Odessa" was nearing the end of her back workout and was seated on the row machine, gasping for air like a fish out of water. Just then, some knucklehead in a tank top (in Brooklyn they call them "wife-beaters") came strutting over.

"How long are duh personal training sessions?" Wife Beater asked.

"An hour," I replied, a little annoyed with the interruption.

"An hour?" he scoffed. "That's it? I train for three! (*pronounced: "tree"*)

"No, you train for 20 minutes," I said. "You spend the rest of the time flapping with your buddies. I've seen you." I glanced at my exhausted client, who was deliriously happy with this unexpected respite.

"Odessa. How long is an hour?"

Odessa swiveled her head in the guy's direction. She was pale, hunched, and sucking air like she just competed in a triathlon, with her sweat-soaked hair hanging in her face like wet spaghetti. "*Trust* me . . . an *hour* . . . is a *long* time!"

Wife Beater's eyes popped. "Yeesh . . ." he said as he turned and walked away.

"Have a nice day, pal."

CHARACTER SPOTLIGHT: ANGRY MEMBER BOB

Over the years, I've learned that most gyms have at least one or two members who are on the aggressive side. I call them Angry Members. You've probably seen them before. They make loud, growling noises or scream while doing sets, drop or toss weights left and right, glare evilly at anyone considering sharing a machine with them, and train with such fury that you wonder if they've ever considered therapy.

When I was a PT at Caveat Sports, I had a favorite Angry Member. Let's call him "Bob." Bob was a skinny, withdrawn teenager who always kept his head down. He was kind of nerdy and had a lot of pent-up anger. I could tell he'd been bullied a lot as a child, so I couldn't help feeling sorry for him.

Bob's problem was that he used to get into violent arguments. Not with other members – with the weight machines. Yes, that's right, inanimate pieces of exercise equipment. He usually picked the ones designed for seated upper body exercises with high, padded backrests. At first, I thought it was because they bore something of a resemblance to a person. I eventually realized it was because they were easier to hit.

Bob's conflicts began with him cursing loudly at the offending machine; soon he'd start whaling away on it. After a round or two, his anger spent, he'd walk quietly away and resume his workout, oblivious to the nervous glances of assorted members and staff.

One day, I was in the middle of training my client, Odessa. We made our way to the seated triceps extension machine. To my consternation, there was Bob, doing sets on the exact machine we needed. He was using about half of the machine's weight stack, and I knew us being there would be a problem for his fragile ego. The weight he was lifting was the same as Odessa's warm-up weight.

In an effort to avoid upsetting Bob, I tried to hang back and wait for him to finish. As luck would have it, he noticed us and chivalrously invited us to work in.

I counted down on the weight stack Bob was using and reduced the weight by five pounds so that Odessa could do her warm-up set. She pumped out an easy twenty reps and got up. Bob walked back over – his chest swollen with pride – and made a big show of counting back down the weight stack. He put the pin back to where it had been previously, pushed out nine or ten reps, and then got off.

Dreading what was coming next, I took a deep breath and put the pin all the way at the bottom (Odessa was so strong at this point she could press the entire rack). Bob staggered in disbelief.

"*She's* gonna do *that*?" he sputtered.

"Watch and learn," I replied.

As he gaped in astonishment, Odessa sat down and blasted out twelve clean reps with the entire stack, smiled girlishly, and got up like it was nothing. Poor Bob was so upset that he squeaked like a frightened squirrel and ran right out of the gym.

I never saw Bob again, which was a darn shame. In all my days, I've never saw *anyone* slug it out with a Nautilus machine the way he did.

CHAPTER 3:

THE TIP OF THE SWORD

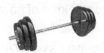

After working as a trainer at Caveat Sports for a year, I was promoted to the position of Training Coordinator.

As the Coordinator, I got a tiny taste of what it meant to have a little power. My salary increased slightly, as did my per-session rates, and I was given authority over the floor instructors and personal trainers at my club.

Beyond that, however, things pretty much stayed the same. I still had to answer to my club's Manager and Assistant Manager, as well as the Floor Manager. Although my increased responsibilities were negligible, I got some additional insight on the innermost workings of my club.

What I discovered wasn't pretty.

HOOKED ON PT – ADDICTION PRINCIPLES

The first thing my company's Area Fitness Manager taught me was how to teach my trainers to get their clients addicted to PT.

Unlike recreational drugs like heroin and cocaine, which enslave the mind and destroy the body, most people don't look at exercise, and personal training in particular, as having the potential to be dangerously addictive.

It can be.

Remember, personal trainers are in the business of making money. Whether they believe in the product they're selling or not, they make their living off the money they rake in from their respective clients. They don't want a client who's only going to do a single session. Flash-in-the-pan clients leave empty hours that must be filled. Trainers want someone who'll stick around – someone who will book two, three, or even five sessions per week, and renew those sessions like clockwork. That's the ideal client.

I was shown many tricks to get clients hooked. And it all starts with our free, introductory session.

Always keep in mind that introductory training sessions are *not* set up to teach you as much as possible. They're designed to draw you in, to hook you on your trainer's knowledge and ability to motivate – and to make you feel utterly dependent, as if without them you'd never accomplish anything.

Of all the places I worked during my twenty years, I think Empirical Sports was the most driven at playing this kind of game. Over time, I watched them reduce their free sessions from two hours to one, then to a single, thirty-minute workout. When that wasn't producing enough conversions, they started offering discount training packages with fancy names like "Fast-Fit" and "Try-N-Train." When they realized their trainers weren't good at selling, they got professional salespeople to make the pitches, and gave them a commission, too.

In the end, it's all about getting deeper into your wallet. I blame the clubs, not the trainers. Most trainers are hoping to change people's lives, not turn them upside down and shake them by their ankles. Unfortunately, they make peanuts if they aren't doing paid sessions. And without paying clients, they can't survive. Some clubs don't pay them anything *except* when they train clients, so you can imagine the position this puts them in.

Given these kinds of incentives, many trainers become very good at waging psychological warfare on their clients. If a client has plateaued (hasn't lost anything from the previous week), the trainer starts asking them about their diet. They find out about that black-and-white cookie their client snuck out of the fridge in the middle of the night, or the large popcorn they shared at the movies the previous weekend.

An eye roll from a "disappointed" trainer can be devastating to a distraught client. It's like your mother scolding you when you're five years old; all you can do is stare at the floor and try not to cry.

My Area Fitness Manager actually told me to "not show my clients too much," to "hold things back," and leak knowledge in "little dribs and drabs." I hated doing this, but in the end I had no choice. I was under pressure from above. I had quotas to hit – both the clubs' and my own – and bills to pay.

I learned how to play with my clients' heads to keep them interested. I'd vary their workouts a little each week by throwing in something new – maybe a slight variant on an existing exercise. I watched them suck up these tiny morsels; they regarded me as a well of infinite knowledge, whose depths they'd just started to explore. A drug addict needs something with a little extra kick every so often, just to keep them drooling.

Not exactly what I thought I'd be doing for my clients when I started.

SURVIVAL TIP #3

A word to the wise about those introductory PT packages: always remember that they're a total set-up. Sure, five sessions for $200 sounds like a bargain. It is – it's only $40 per workout. You may think that's all you need, but your trainer has other ideas.

There's always more to learn. And your trainer will constantly remind you of how much more they can do for you if you stick around.

Of course, once your discount package runs out, lo and behold, you get to buy training at regular prices! Suddenly, your $40 per hour rate has jumped to $75! Holy cow, run for the door!

But wait . . . if you take advantage of the big training sale, which is "expiring" that same day, you can buy twenty sessions for only $1,200. That's saving $15 per session. You'll save $300 by acting immediately, and your trainer will be by your side twice a week for the next ten weeks!

Naturally, there's always a sale. So don't be surprised when your twenty sessions are running out and you get a call from your trainer, or even the club manager. Expect to hear about a one-day-only opportunity that will save you a bundle, one that's too good for you to miss.

And so, the cycle continues . . .

POOR HYGIENE

I can't speak for everyone, but *I* wouldn't want to smell like a dead moose. If you can see the stink waves coming off the guy on the machine next to you, then it's time to draw the line. As a trainer, and even as a manager, this was something I had to deal with on a regular basis.

We live in an age of soap and indoor plumbing. You'd think this type of thing wouldn't be an issue. It is. Some people go to the gym excessively dolled up (or even train in high heels – they're called peacocks), but there are just as many people who don't care how they look (or smell). They skip showers, deodorant, and laundry, neither knowing nor caring that you and I are struggling not to lose our lunch.

It's easy to tell when someone really smells. No matter how crowded the gym is, they will always have an array of empty machines around them – like an invisible force field. Maybe that's why they never wash: they know they can always get free equipment.

I've seen some facility owners – typically in small bodybuilding gyms – sniff out the offending party like a bloodhound. Once he discovered the perpetrator, the owner would politely tell them, "You stink. Get the fuck out – and don't come back until you take a shower!"

Naturally, most of the bigger chains won't risk such effective measures. They'd rather hold their noses and pretend the problem doesn't exist.

When I was a floor instructor at Caveat Sports, there was a European woman there who wore the same exact outfit, day after day and week after week. She smelled like horribly spoiled milk. And nobody had the decency to let her know she had a problem, they just mocked her behind her back. The running joke was that – after she peeled it off – her workout suit stood up all on its own and waited for her in her closet.

Then there was this Russian guy. He was huge, almost seven feet tall. The staff used to call him "Chernobyl." Let me tell you, that European girl smelled bad up close, but this guy reeked from twenty feet away. His body odor was so pungent it seemed like he'd smeared rotting onions in his armpits.

One day, Chernobyl was training hard. This particular gym had a small running track that encircled its main floor, and in between each weight set he'd run a lap. His odor, combined with the club's sub-standard air conditioning, resulted in a vortex of stench that made breathing impossible. I watched, horrified, as my members fled en masse to find fresh air.

Finally fed up, my floor manager told me to go tell Chernobyl that he should leave – or at least take a shower. I was with a client, so I refused (actually, my client wanted me to do it as well, but I figured I'd get in a fight and get fired). My boss pulled rank and ordered me to enter the noxious cloud. I eventually complied, but in retrospect, I question her wisdom. At the time, I wasn't exactly known for my tact.

I walked up to Chernobyl, prepared for anything, and crooked a finger at him. "I need a word with you," I said.

He stared curiously down at me. "Yes?"

I took a deep breath (and quickly regretted it). "Look . . . I don't know how they do things where *you* come from, but in *this* country we *shower* after our workouts . . ."

"I *do.*" he interjected.

"We use *deodorant* . . ."

"I *do!*"

"And we *wash* our *gym clothes* every time we use them."

"I . . ."

I watched him freeze and knew I'd hit the bull's-eye. He was against the ropes, and I went in for the kill. "You see, there've been some complaints. Because, frankly, you stink! I'm afraid I'm going to have to ask you to leave, and please don't come back until this problem has been rectified."

Completely mortified, Chernobyl left the club looking quite a bit smaller than when he came in. I never saw him again. I suppose he was too ashamed to come back. I felt really bad about what I'd done, even if it was my boss's fault.

Oh well . . . pass the Right Guard!

NOW *THAT'S* CLASS

During my years in the industry, I've interacted with hundreds of personal trainers. Their personalities and work ethics varied. Some were eminently professional, some lackadaisical, and some outright insane.

Being naïve and admittedly chauvinistic, I used to think that female trainers would somehow be different than the guys. I assumed that, because they were women, they'd be nicer, classier, and with higher moral standards.

Boy was *I* an idiot.

After meeting trainers of both sexes, I was surprised to discover that the girls were just as bad. Sometimes they were worse. I was also stunned to discover that many of them took steroids – a few even bragged about it. In some cases, this might have accounted for their exaggerated mood swings, as well as their hyper-muscularity and overt sexuality.

Back when I was working at Empirical Sports, I knew a trainer named "Dusky" who was a fitness competitor. Judging by her physique and husky voice – not to mention that she repeatedly got into fights over parking spots – Dusky was definitely on the juice. She had problems holding onto a man. She used to come to me constantly for relationship advice (why, I have *no* idea) and changed boyfriends almost weekly.

One day, Dusky came into my office while I was chatting with a friend. Out of nowhere, she offered us both a threesome. We were stunned, to say the least. When I refused, she changed tactics and offered me one-on-one casual sex, "no strings attached," behind my girl's back, whenever it was "mutually convenient." And, of course, no one would ever know.

As Dusky was telling me all this, I pictured her walking around my club the week before, showing off horrendous bite marks that decorated both her thighs. She looked like a shark attack victim. Half the gym heard about how the bruises were from "rough sex."

I decided to pass on Dusky's generous offer. I was well aware of the creature I'd become. Why would I want to hook up with the female version of myself?

CHARACTER SPOTLIGHT: "SORE" LOSER

I'd barely recovered from the aforementioned incident, when another trainer offered me a threesome. Her name was "Amazing," and she was scarier than Dusky by far. She was a bodybuilder. Take away the lipstick and eye shadow, and she was a solid mass of muscle without an ounce of fat on her. Don't get me wrong; I am sure there are plenty of men out there into women bigger and stronger than they are. I'm just not one of them.

Amazing walked brazenly into my office and plopped down in a chair. She leaned far back, intertwining her arms above her head until her triple-D silicone breasts strained her sports bra to the absolute max. Once she figured she had my full attention, she made some small talk. Then, out of nowhere, she asked, "So, when are you taking me to dinner?"

"Excuse me? Don't you have a boyfriend?"

"Yes, but he won't mind."

My jaw dropped. "I see . . . well, you *do* know I'm in a relationship, right?"

She gave me a seductive look and said, "So then . . . you can take *both* of us out to dinner."

"*Both* of you?" I echoed.

As she nodded, I felt my ego start to deflate. I realized that it wasn't *me* she was after. Amazing was a notoriously active bisexual and had never shown any interest in me until that point. She was obviously looking to score with the insanely hot woman I'd been seeing. I was just a means to an end, a patsy.

"Are you suggesting what I think you are?" I asked.

"Maybe . . ." she said with a smirk.

"I'll have to get back to you on that."

I shuddered as she left my office. Even if I could have accepted Amazing's motives – and was the least bit interested in her mannish body – the ill-concealed, purple, raisin-shaped sore festering on her upper lip was enough to make anyone run for the hills.

CHARACTER SPOTLIGHT: ROMEO, ROMEO...

Moral rock bottom has to be a guy I knew back at Caveat Sports. This dude (let's refer to him as "Rod") was beyond the pale – and this is coming from *me*.

Rod was a big guy with a great smile, but for some reason he didn't want to date the women at the club where he worked. I thought it might have been because he had a serious girlfriend, or perhaps he was afraid. Regardless, he was up to some very dark and devious "outsourcing."

From what his manager and coworkers told me, Rod ended up getting his hands on a police officer's badge and began scouring the seedier parts of the city for prostitutes. When he found one, he pulled over, flashed his "badge," and made her get in. With his size and shield, the girl was easily convinced he was NYPD. Then he'd pull into the nearest dark alley and give her an ultimatum: either open wide and give him a blowjob or be brought "downtown."

Can you imagine?

Now, I want you to take a minute and think about something – this guy was *training* people. He was doing what trainers do, i.e. grabbing people around the hips while spotting them, holding their legs open while stretching them, leaning over and breathing on them . . .

From what I heard, Rod's NYPD routine lasted for months. Fortunately for society, one of the hookers he'd harassed recognized him from the gym (health clubs do not discriminate) and ratted him out to the *real* cops. A quick sting was set up and poor ol' Rod ended up going to jail.

I imagine it was *his* turn to give blow jobs . . .

ULTERIOR MOTIVES

Based on what I've seen (and done) over the years, I've come to the conclusion that a lot of women hire personal trainers purely to sleep with them.

Sure, I've seen men join gyms because of a hot female trainer on the floor during a tour (it didn't hurt that I fanned the flames of their desire). However, just as many women came into my club purely looking for a trainer to "work on them." A few times I actually caught trainers getting it on with their clients in the club, usually in one of our closets. Sadly, I was forced to fire the trainers and revoke their clients' memberships as well.

After all, it *is* a health club.

I could usually tell when a woman was looking for "one-on-one" sessions because she'd ask to meet all my trainers before she decided to join. She'd look them over and gravitate toward whichever one she found the most appealing (big muscles, heavy jaw, rippling abs . . .). Then, there were certain inevitable questions she'd ask me about the trainer during the enrollment process ("How old is he? Does he go to school? Is he married or seeing someone?"). A few women even told me their girlfriend recommended a particular trainer after working with him "personally."

If I ever doubted my suspicions, a few questions (on the down-low, of course) to the trainer in question usually confirmed things. One guy I worked with used to take his client to a nearby motel during his lunch break (with her paying, naturally). Another got a ride home from his client each night (to *her* home, not his). And still another bragged to me about how he banged his clients in the backseat of his car, after work, right down the street from the club.

Frankly, what people do outside of work is their business. What bothered me was that most of these women were married – many of them "happily." They usually had kids and husbands with lots of money, but they were bored and their needs obviously weren't being met. Rather than finding an escort, they opted for a somewhat safer and more practical approach. I suppose it was a smart move. I'm sure my guys gave them good workouts.

To be sure, on those occasions that a husband found out and came storming into the club, things *did* get a little complicated.

Editor's Note: It pays to have planned escape routes for your trainers – out the side door, through the alley, over the fence . . .

SURVIVAL TIP #4

I once read a survey that said the most likely place for people to meet someone for an affair is at a health club. And the second most likely person they'll have that affair with is their personal trainer.

So, if your significant other is joining a gym, be aware of the sexual minefield they're walking into. Trainers are typically lean and fit, with enviable physiques and entertaining personalities. They work very closely with their clients – getting to know them, listening to their stories and complaints, encouraging them in their efforts. Trainers might even hear about their client's relationship problems.

For the guys out there, let me paint an unpleasant picture: your girl just finished working with her stud of a trainer, who stood behind her the entire time, holding her hips while she did deep squats and encouraging her to "push hard." Now she's lying on a mat, on her back; he's on top of her, stretching her in a position that belongs in an adult film. She's breathing hard, she's sweaty, her adrenaline is pumping, and this big, built man that she enjoys spending time with is straddling her – his crotch only inches away.

What do you think is going through her mind?

And ladies, don't think you're off the hook. When your man goes to the gym, he'll run into scores of women looking for "gym buddies." And the sexually charged female trainers are just as ravenous – if not more so – than the guys . . .

So take my advice. If your partner is going to be working with a trainer – unless you have a textbook-perfect relationship and the confidence of Brad Pitt – keep both eyes open.

Oh, and to answer your obvious question, the most likely person for your significant other to have an affair with (according to that same survey) is the health club salesperson who signed them up.

Did I mention I went into sales after I gave up being a PT?

CHAPTER 4:

PERSONAL TRAINING SURVIVAL GUIDE

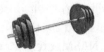

To train or not to train?

You've finally joined a gym. You've made a major step and should be congratulated. But now there's a question to consider: should you invest in hiring a fitness professional, or simply go it on your own? A workout with a qualified personal trainer is four times as effective as one on your own, but is it something *you* really need?

If you're a former athlete or had five years of gym experience under your belt before becoming a couch potato, a trainer might not be necessary. Most of the equipment is still the same. If a quick crash course on the newest machines is all you need, then a single session may be enough to get you back on track. On the other hand, if you have little or no experience working out, multiple sessions with a trainer is a more *pressing* notion.

Of all the places I worked, only one chain, Dinar Fitness, gave three legitimate sessions to each new client. Not surprisingly, their members exercised more and were more physically fit. On the other hand, places like Caveat Sports, which gave only one session, had members who got poorer results. A few days after signing them up, I'd see confused newbies wandering around the gym. I watched as they engaged in what I call "monkey-see, monkey-do" style training: they'd see someone with an admirable physique and try to imitate their workout, whether it was safe or not.

The second thing to consider when looking at a potential trainer is their qualifications. Do they specialize in the area you want to improve (Weight loss, bodybuilding, core training, etc.)? Are they certified? Believe it or not, many health clubs (including most of the ones I worked at) will hire anyone who wants to be a trainer, as long as they're in shape and management thinks they can make some money. But just because someone looks good doesn't mean they know what they're doing. Some people are naturally athletic and can look great doing pushups and eating cupcakes. That doesn't mean their fitness routine will work for anyone else.

Larger fitness chains usually offer their own certification course (which they charge their trainers for, naturally). It also helps them legally (in the event of a training mishap) and limits the trainer's options to work elsewhere – rival health clubs will turn their noses up at a competitor's certification. Top trainers know this and try to get certified by more prestigious national organizations (ACE, NASM, etc.). Many are certified three or four times over. Trainers also tend to have some background in nutrition, with a few even being full-fledged dieticians.

The last thing to consider is price, and of course your budget. PT is far from cheap, and some clients spend a grand or more a month on packages. A word to the wise: always keep in mind that health clubs make major money off personal training. And that cash often goes right in the owners' pockets. Once you invest in a large session package, management will automatically target you as a potential cash cow. They will try to milk you, and often. If you only plan to do the sessions you bought, tell them up front, and be direct about it.

Otherwise, be prepared to have some very sore nipples.

CHARACTER SPOTLIGHT: CORPORAL PUNISHMENT

The most brutal trainer I ever saw worked at U.S. Amazing Fitness. He was a real gung-ho type, fresh out of the Marine Corps. Let's call him "Corporal Punishment," or "CP" for short.

Although CP seemed like a good fit at first, within a week I realized he was *way* too hardcore to work in a health club. I watched him get in his clients' faces and scream at them like a drill sergeant at Paris Island. Any perceived slacking was met with abusive punishment, just like in basic training. Besides his intimidation tactics, CP's boot camp-style training techniques were dangerous, and I worried that sooner or later he was going to hurt someone.

I talked to CP about lightening up, but it was pointless. He wouldn't listen to anyone, least of all me. But soon he did something I couldn't ignore. He was working with a young lady I'd signed up the day before: a petite blonde, maybe five feet tall and a hundred pounds. He had her strapped into a leg extension machine loaded up with so much weight that when she tried straightening her legs, it hoisted her up and out of the seat.

To make matters worse, each time she catapulted up, CP grabbed her by the shoulders and shoved her roughly back down, screaming, "Three more! I want three more!" in her ear.

To her credit, the girl did her best, but it was more than she could handle. I saw her grimace and clutch at her leg. She tried to climb off the machine, but cried out as her knee buckled. She eventually got her bearings and limped toward the locker room, leaning on a nearby wall for support. The whole time her trainer followed her, yelling, "Did I say you could quit? C'mon, walk it off!"

I was horrified. I couldn't believe I stood by and watched CP injure someone. I approached him about it afterward, but I couldn't get through to him. He was too obsessed with his self-image as a trained killer – the one that he planned molding others into.

I had no choice after that. I went to the owners and told them what happened, and about the lawsuit that was undoubtedly heading our way. A day later, they fired Corporal Punishment. Fearing retaliation from their would-be Rambo, they blamed his termination on me. And I was fine with that. The guy was going to get someone killed. Something had to be done.

The next day, CP called me on the phone and tried threatening me. I told him to go scratch his ass. A few years later, he showed up at my job at Dinar Fitness, looking for work. As soon as he saw me he knew his chances of getting a job there were nil. Due to a series of surgeries, I'd gotten out of shape – especially compared to my usual physique. He mouthed off at me in front of my colleagues.

"I see you put on some weight," he said with a smirk.

I gave him a humorless smile. "Yes, I did. But I can lose weight. You'll *always* be an asshole."

Corporal Punishment's smirk vanished. Jaw clenched, he stormed out of my club, muttering to himself.

I guess he preferred dishing out punishment over taking it . . .

TOO MUCH REPETITION

This section isn't about how many sets or reps you should do, or even how many days you hit the gym. It addresses the boredom a personal trainer faces when working with clients. It's more or less inevitable. They see the same people, day in and day out, sometimes with minimal rewards for their efforts.

First and foremost, trainers get worn out because of money. Even if they had loftier goals when they first started (I did), the constant pressure to meet quota brings out their mercenary side. They start viewing clients less as people and more like wads of cash. And they end up only wanting to train those who'll keep paying.

Clients pick up on this. Have you ever joined a gym and met a trainer that seemed all gung ho to work with you, only to watch them deflate like a leaky balloon once they realized you weren't buying a package?

Boredom and disappointment are also major factors. Some clients buy package after package but fail to make progress, no matter how hard they train. Whether they're sneaking into the fridge late at night or canceling sessions, these clients give you a hopeless feeling: one step forward, two steps back.

Some of my colleagues have complained that they feel more like therapists than personal trainers. It happens. When I was a trainer, my clients unloaded all sorts of emotional baggage on me (the lousy boyfriend, the cheating husband, the stalking ex, etc.). It wore me out after a while.

The last six months I was a trainer, I refused to re-up most of my clients. I was determined to change my image and make my job more rewarding: I would only work with beautiful women. And I pulled it off. Within a month I was training ten of the most gorgeous girls in the gym.

Believe it or not, hot babes are easier to sell PT to than other people. Often, they're so insecure about their looks that they'll jump at the opportunity to work with someone who'll tell them how to get even better. And most trainers (like the men who wish they could date such women, but fear to hit on them) are too intimidated to approach them. This leaves them an untapped resource, just waiting for someone like me.

When I worked at Empirical Sports one of my favorite trainers was a guy named "Daniel." He was one of the best I've ever seen, yet he got sick of the business and quit. And it wasn't because he was tired of his clients or the pressure (admittedly, he did complain about an elderly client who farted on him every time she did a set). He gave up personal training because he was disgusted with the corporate culture.

A new District Manager had taken over our region. He was one of those people who tries to clean house after taking the helm. He decided that Daniel had been there "too long" and wanted to fire him at the first opportunity. The fact that Daniel was professional, reliable, and had a great physique meant nothing. So when he missed quota one time, the DM was all over him like a cheap suit.

I went to bat for Daniel and kept him from getting canned, but he was so disgusted by the experience I knew it was just a matter of time before he moved on to greener pastures. Frankly, I can't blame him.

On the bright side, at least he let me sign him up for a membership a few weeks before he tendered his resignation.

LOOKING GOOD CAN COST YOU

One thing I was surprised to discover as a personal trainer was how unscrupulous my peers could be. I was amazed by how many of them cheated the system. Just to start with, a big percentage of them took money under the table from their clients, instead of channeling it through the club and getting paid their fair share.

You might wonder why this problem is so widespread.

Based on my experience, health club owners are greedy and don't take care of their people. A session with a professional personal trainer typically starts at $60 per hour (some are twice that). But the club takes anywhere from 50-65% of that fee, leaving the trainer making peanuts. It's far from fair. Personal training is hard work; throwing weights around and working with clients takes a lot of physical and mental effort. If you do thirty sessions each week and make only $600 – while your employer pockets $1200 and treats you like garbage – you're not going to be very happy.

Taking money under the table is chancy. There are career-threatening ramifications if a trainer gets caught. The first trainer I saw get busted (and fired on the spot) was a dude from my certification class. This genius asked a brand-new client to make out a big, fat check for PT in *his* name, instead of the club's. The member, understandably suspicious, went to the club manager and asked if that was the norm.

Unemployment line, there he blows!

Naturally, most trainers aren't that brazen (or brainless), and they'll usually try to establish a bond with their client first. They become close, like a bartender and a barfly, but with the benefits of improved health instead of necrosis of the liver. Once a level of trust is established, the trainer offers the client to work with them off the books. The trainer will make more (say $45 off the books instead of $20 on) and the client pays less.

The risk of getting caught also decreases dramatically. The client usually empathizes with their trainer. They want to help their unappreciated fitness guru by forming an alliance with them against *the man,* aka the evil gym owner.

Of course, given my vulnerability to temptation, topped off by my need to support my "extreme dating" (*can I copyright that?*), it was just a matter of time before I jumped on the band wagon and started pocketing cash, too. But, believe me, I had no intention of getting caught like all those guys I'd seen come and go.

At Caveat Sports, it was surprisingly easy. Back then, we sold clients coupon booklets of PT sessions and turned in one for each completed workout. My manager trusted me implicitly, so it was a simple matter to accept chunks of cash from my most loyal clientele and keep a few coupons in reserve, just in case. No one kept tabs on the exact number of sessions being done anyway, and if anyone ever questioned me, I simply said, "Yes, but he's got to renew soon. He's down to his last three. See?"

Editor's Note: It's like carrying condoms – you may not be <u>*expecting*</u> *to get screwed, but it's good to be prepared.*

SURVIVAL TIP #5

For those of you currently working with a personal trainer "under the table" or considering it, a word to the wise: If you get caught your trainer will be instantly fired. You may or may not be thrown out of the gym (you probably won't; companies will typically say it was the trainer's fault for misleading you – they still want your money).

To make matters worse, the gym is under no obligation to give you back your cash. And, I guarantee the trainer you prepaid sure as heck won't (prepare yourself for: "Sorry, I already spent it."). So, unless your cash-and-carry trainer has facilities at home where they can complete your training package, or you're willing to follow them to another gym, look before you leap.

If you don't, at the very least invest in small packages. That way it'll be less painful cutting your losses when the shit hits the fan.

CHAPTER 5:

THE MOVE TO SALES

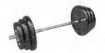

After working as a trainer for some eighteen months, I came to the uncomfortable realization that the income I was pulling in from Caveat Sports had reached its ceiling. With my company consuming 2/3 of what I earned for each paid session, I was only making $20 a workout. Even at a full forty sessions per week, that amounted to only $800 per week, or approximately 40K per year. Pretty lousy compensation for all the work I was doing, I decided.

Sure, I pulled in some extra money under the table, but that was about it. And training that many sessions per week was hard. I just wasn't making enough green to justify continuing the job.

Many of my colleagues and clients told me that I should consider moving into sales. Initially, I railed against the idea – even though I heard it was where the money was. I despised pushy salespeople. Plus, after seeing our Area Manager, Johnson, abusing his staff, and knowing I'd be answering to him, I was hardly interested. You can imagine my surprise when I found out that my manager was making the company average of 85K year – more than double my salary. And doing sales was the fast track to management. Can you blame me for having a change of heart?

I called Johnson and told him I was looking to make the move. I expected him to resist, but to my surprise, he was quite amenable to me changing gears. Maybe he knew how well I sold PT and trusted me to sell memberships; more likely, he still held a grudge and wanted me under his thumb so he could exact revenge.

Either way, I wasn't about to complain. I'd seen the sales reps at my club "working." They didn't. Ninety percent of the time they sat around joking in their offices or yakking on the phone. There was no running around the gym, no loading and unloading 45 lb. weight plates, no cheerleading or tear-drying. Selling was easy work that paid well, and I knew once I was the boss, I'd make a killing.

Without another word – or thought to the perils that might await me – I bequeathed my collection of hotties to those trainers I deemed worthy (I kept a *few* ladies to train off duty – more on that later) and jumped ship without so much as a "fare-thee-well."

"Bring on those fat, juicy commissions, people. Manager's chair, here I come!"

GIMME YOUR MONEY

"It pays to know your enemy."

Those were the first words of advice I received from our Regional Director when I underwent sales training at Caveat Sports.

When I first started pushing gym memberships, I was gentle, even mellow. I had no formal training when it came to selling and disliked that whole "used car salesman" image. I told my clients that I was a personal trainer, not a salesman. It made them lower their guard a bit; they focused more on discussing training. Actual membership pricing became a secondary consideration, which made the closing portion of my sales easier. By the time we reached the price presentation, my clients just wanted to get it over with and start their workouts.

Once I went through sales training, however, my presentations changed – and not for the better. I wasn't used to looking at potential customers as "the enemy." ("Those bastards each have $50 of your money in their back pocket that you need to get back.") Nor was I accustomed to using hard-closing sales tactics or playing mental chess.

After going through my company's sales training, I actually had a harder time selling, and my numbers dropped instead of climbing. I tried to do things their way and become someone I'm not. I was faking it and came across as robotic and grasping.

Not a good thing.

After some pondering, I shrugged off the bulk of my company's sales training. I used Bruce Lee's kung fu principles, absorbing what was useful and disregarding what wasn't. Eventually, the company got what they wanted: I came out of my shell and turned into the cold-blooded selling machine they wanted me to be.

It could have been the pressure they put me (and all salespeople) under, or maybe it was just the allure of money. Probably both. Regardless, I changed. The "good guy" trainer vanished and a new Max emerged – greedy and calloused. If someone wasn't about to pull out their wallet, I wouldn't give them the time of day. What did I care about their problems? I had quotas to hit. I needed commissions!

In retrospect, my reptilian womanizing tendencies must have finally bled over into my selling. My original fear that stopped me from becoming a veterinarian – losing my humanity and not caring whether animals lived or died – had caught up with me. When I looked at people as they walked through the door, I no longer saw human beings that needed my help.

I only saw money.

My favorite victims were unsuspecting immigrants with less-than-perfect English, be they Chinese, Arabic or Russian. It was a habit I picked up from Robert. But instead of cracking jokes at their expense, I robbed them blind. I greeted my prey at the door and psychologically ran them over like a freight train.

It was easy to do. I was intimidating to begin with, being over six feet tall and heavily muscled. I'd smile, give them a crushing handshake, and then lead them into my office. After guiding them into the hot seat, I loomed over them. Our conversation usually went something like this:

"Okay, "John," it's your lucky day. You've hit the jackpot! I've got the sale of the year going on, today only! Our membership is three full years at every club for only $959, and after that it's only $99 per year. Isn't that great?"

Before John could say anything I'd cut him off and ask, "What credit card do you have with you?"

"Um, a . . . Visa?"

I'd smile again. The poor bastard had fallen into my trap. Still standing over him, I'd nod and say, "Great! Let me see it."

At this point, John actually opened his wallet and handed me his credit card. I snatched it from him, swiped it through, and printed his contract and receipt while he was still wondering what the heck was going on. I didn't even *ask* if he wanted to join or give him membership options. I just handed him his contract, showed him where to sign, handed him his copy and membership card, then shook his trembling hand and hoisted him back out of the seat.

Congratulating him on his wise purchase, I guided John back out the door, telling him his trainer would call in a few days for an appointment. It was unbelievable. The entire process took 3-4 minutes at most, and my receptionist would stare in disbelief as my new "member" staggered outside and down the street in a stupor, a contract in one hand and still-smoking credit card in the other.

Believe it or not, I used this technique on scores of people, and it rarely failed. To be honest, I had no idea if they ever *used* the gym, but I didn't care. All that mattered was that I got paid.

Editor's Note: I don't know if there's a hell for salespeople. But if there is, I'm sure my office will have a view . . .

SALES 101

Salespeople look at you as the enemy. They will exploit you, and any psychological weaknesses you may have, to make you do what they want, i.e., give them your hard-earned cash.

Why shouldn't you have the same advantage?

I'm going to teach you all about health club sales and the people that promote them, so that you know *exactly* what you're dealing with. I'll give you an in-depth look at how the sales process works, from generating business on down, and show you where a rep is coming from in terms of technique, goals, and even motivation. And share some personal stories along the way . . .

COMPENSATION

Cash, cabbage, bucks, greenbacks . . . *MONEY*. Call it what you will, everything revolved around money back when I worked in memberships. And I guarantee you, absolutely nothing has changed.

Salespeople in the fitness industry are motivated by two factors: greed and fear. The greed part is pretty straightforward. They want money – your money. A sales rep makes money in the gym in the following ways:

- *Salary. Gym salaries are notoriously small – especially for the sales staff. This is done deliberately to make them work as hard as possible – hence making the company more money. Most salaries are minimum wage (if that), with some even based on a "draw on commission" system. Bloodthirsty competition and constant in-fighting keeps the staff at each other's throats – and also makes them more apt to act dishonestly.*

- **Commissions.** *The core of a sales rep's paycheck. Commissions on gym memberships vary from company to company and membership to membership. As a rule of thumb, the more expensive the gym, the bigger the commission, from as little as $5.00-$10.00 to as much as $100.00-$200.00. Obviously, the more expensive the plan, the bigger the commission. Hence, the salesperson will always push the priciest plan first, then downgrade to adapt to the prospect's level of resistance. Salespeople often get paid for added services, such as personal training, massage, nutrition plans, and even tanning. They always try to up-sell.*
- **Bonuses.** *Most health clubs offer their sales staff a bonus if they meet or exceed their quota. This may take the form of a set dollar amount: if you go 10% over quota you get "X" dollars, more at 20% over, etc. Some also offer a bonus per sale. Often the best time to join a gym ((if you're looking for a deal) is the last day or two of the month. Salespeople who are close to hitting quota will bend over backwards to get your business. Just make sure you're really getting everything they promise you.*

Quotas are also where the fear factor comes in. Club managers, and those they answer to, take their membership quotas very seriously. And anyone lower down on the food chain who fails to produce will find themselves in the crosshairs.

Gym sales reps are under constant pressure. If they falter, they *will* be disciplined. Their supervisor might initially chew them out, but things escalate very quickly into write-ups, suspensions, and eventually, termination (usually without unemployment benefits).

With all that hanging over their heads, plus their innate competitiveness and greed, reps will say or do anything to hit their numbers. I suppose I should have never been surprised by the things I saw go down . . .

CHARACTER SPOTLIGHT: ALL DOLLARS, NO SENSE

When I first started doing sales, I was forced to compete with an older gentleman who was a little on the eccentric side. We'll refer to him as "Dillinger." Dillinger had some interesting character traits. He was obsessed with a fitness product he'd concocted – one he claimed had absolutely no manufacturing costs and would make a ton of money in the direct response market.

One day, he showed me his invention. He handed me a wadded-up ball of some strange, fibrous material. He claimed it was a new hand exerciser that would set the market on fire. When I noted that it didn't seem to provide any resistance, he explained to me that it was made out of dog hair, shed from his poodle.

I looked closely at what I was holding in my hand, and – to my horror – I could see fleas crawling and jumping around.

In addition to his other quirks, Dillinger was very devious. He took advantage of my inexperience with sales, and pulled out all the stops to win our club's coveted monthly bonus. His duplicity was without end. He'd lurk behind the front desk ("hawking" it), answering the phone for the receptionist and sneaking sales calls. He also used some annoying tactics, telling my clients things like: "Oh, he's not in today. But he can see you tomorrow, if you like." ("Tomorrow," of course, was my day off.) Or my personal favorite, "He doesn't work here anymore. No, he died . . . Yes, it was very tragic . . ."

This went on for weeks. Being a neophyte, I had no experience dealing with this type of treachery, so I didn't know what to do. Eventually, I got mad. With my manager on vacation and nowhere else to turn, I went to Johnson, our Area Manager, and told him what was happening. He laughed and told me he "loved stuff like that." In his mind it fostered a more competitive work environment and generated more business.

Having gotten no justice from Johnson, my relationship with Dillinger continued to sour. Eventually, I outright hated the guy. Undaunted, he kept stealing my hard-earned business – sometimes right under my nose.

Things finally came to a head. I was standing outside the sales offices, when Dillinger came barreling down the hallway at full speed. Although he had plenty of room to pass, he decided to come right at me. My back was turned, and all I heard him say was, "Outta the way, fool!" as he gave me a violent shove. I was sent pitching face-first into the hallway's carpeted drywall.

My temper exploded; with murder in my eyes, I hauled back and threw a vicious haymaker at the back of Dillinger's head. He was moving at a good clip, and his velocity saved him. I missed him by inches, and he never knew until I told him months later.

It was probably a good thing. At the very least, I'd have gotten fired. Still, it just goes to show, you can only push someone so far.

Oh, and for the record, I won that bonus.

QUOTAS

When it comes to building a gym's membership base, it's a case of shoveling sand against the tide. Once a club hits saturation (the point where everyone has to wait 30 minutes or more for a treadmill), growth is maxed out. Sales then are mostly made to replenish the endless parade of cancelations all clubs experience.

No one stays at a gym forever. People move, get hurt or pregnant, or decide life is better as a couch potato. Whatever the case, quotas are put in place to offset this perpetual fiscal bleeding. They're how gyms stay in business and why their sales guys don't just sit around with their thumbs up their proverbial butts and check out hot babes. (Okay, sales guys do that anyways, but at least the company knows they'll make some money in the process).

If you *don't* hit your quota, there will be penalties. Some companies will cut off your non-generated traffic (guests and walk-ins) until you start pulling your weight. Of course, that makes it even harder to do your job.

Others will just fire you.

Regardless, the tremendous pressure health clubs put on their staff leads to some very interesting inter-personal dynamics.

CHARACTER SPOTLIGHT: MARK THE SHARK

A favorite sales colleague of mine at Empirical Sports was a guy we'll refer to as "Mark." Mark was great: laid back, funny, and always there to help out a friend. His only flaw was that he was a former drug dealer who'd done a lengthy stretch in prison.

In fitness, the bosses usually don't bother doing background checks – which contributes mightily to the industry's high turnover rate. It also means that you may have had a drug dealer (or worse) sell you your gym membership.

Despite his pharmaceutical sales experience, Mark wasn't very good at selling memberships. Dissatisfied with his salary and commissions, he decided to do something about it. Why settle for $75 per sale when you can make $500? His solution was ingenious: he found and exploited a loophole in the computer system.

The company's membership system was set up so that thirty-day guest passes could be entered for promotions and barter exchanges. Aware of this, Mark told people, "The gym is normally $1,000 per year. You give me $500 cash, and I'll give you the whole year!"

People were jumping at it.

The scam worked well. All Mark had to keep adding thirty-day extensions for his people and no one was the wiser. He was cleaning up. Just four of those a week was two grand in his pocket. Mark only got caught after he was transferred to another location. He never kept a hit list of all his "clients," and was unable to keep track of their extensions. Once the "memberships" started coming up expired at the front desk, it came to light that they weren't actual members – just guests being given a free (or reduced) ride. Naturally, when they insisted they paid cash for the year, it was obvious something was going on. The manager got involved and the jig was up; poor Mark was fired.

Every cloud has a silver lining: I got to sign up a good percentage of his clients.

Mark was not, by *any* means, the only one gaming the system. With my front desk on full-time alert for *any* thirty-day pass, we stopped everyone and checked them all. Scores of them were fraudulent. The con men soon adapted and became more sophisticated. They discovered they could put an expiration date in the computer that the system wouldn't recognize – say, a thirty-day pass ending a full three years later. Once we found out, my manager informed tech-support; a quick change eliminated the glitch.

The criminals evolved again. They started operating outside their clubs. They'd work the street corners of NYC like hookers, offering people rates of $500 for one year or $800 for two. People familiar with our real rates were like: "Wow, what a bargain!"

Once the con artist had his patsy, he would take their cash and send them to a location in another borough to pick up their "membership." An accomplice there would put them in for a thirty-day pass, and if questioned by management, pretended to know nothing. And whoever took the money had long since vanished. They used fake Empirical Sports business cards with an alias on them, and a cell number that could never be traced. It was impossible for the victims to prove anything.

SURVIVAL TIP #6

If you're going to buy a membership using cash, make sure you get a computerized receipt and an official contract. Con men can go to any location where they have a friend working and pretend it's their club.

And for God's sake don't give money to some guy you just met on the street.

If you do get taken and can't prove what occurred, rest assured the company will do nothing. No refund, no credit. Believe me, I know. I saw it happen dozens of times. Some yelled and screamed and kicked up a fuss. And some were psychotic enough to try and get revenge, personally. But all of them ended up losing their money.

Besides con men like Mark, the only people who benefit are the salespeople, who'll exploit the fallout for a nice, easy commission.

CHARACTER SPOTLIGHT: SLIMY AND SLIMIER

Another interesting technique to watch out for was used by two more of my former Empirical Sports co-workers. Let's call them "Joke" and "Waxworth."

Their innovations were eventually picked up by con men throughout the company.

Joke was a sneaky individual who always bothered me for cover stories so he wouldn't get caught cheating on his poor girlfriend. I wouldn't have cared that much, except that he constant bragged about how he'd taken her virginity and then had her paying his rent and bills.

Even I have my limits.

Waxworth was more interesting. He was an extremely religious type who "found salvation" after a life of drugs, cage-dancing in gay bars, and sleeping with strippers. He was just a *little bit* out there. He told me a story once about how a hard-up guy propositioned him in our club sauna. When the guy realized Waxworth wasn't interested he dropped his towel and started rubbing one out right next to him. Instead of cursing him out and reporting him, Waxworth closed his eyes and counted to ninety before he got up and left.

Ninety? Well, to each his own.

Waxworth told me lots of other stories. About how his girl would only have sex with him if he wore fishnets and panties, how she used to pee on him, or the time she shoved a candle up his ass while he slept.

Editor's Note: I hope it was a birthday candle and not one of those big, red votive things from church (ouch!). Come to think of it, he never did say if the damned thing was lit or not . . .

Working in cahoots, Joke and Waxworth developed unique ways of stealing sales. They weren't pocketing money directly, but they definitely found ways to boost their numbers.

The first one was pretty cut and dry. They'd find a member who was paying more than the current special, convince them to cancel, and then re-sign them. This gave them an extra commission – while costing the company money. With many memberships being pay-as-you-go, it was easy to do. They even changed the member's name and address to reduce the risk of getting caught. Unfortunately, once in a while they forgot to cancel the original membership. When the poor member got billed twice he or she would come in crying. Especially after they discovered that the company would hold them responsible for *both* contracts (yes, it's legal). By trying to save a few bucks, the customers ended up paying double.

That's when the trouble started for my two colleagues. For sure, since they were selling machines, the manager wanted them around, so he turned a semi-blind eye to their shenanigans. Occasionally, he even helped cover for them. That is, after giving them a stern warning and threatening them both with a beating.

Their second technique turned out to be a little harder to cover up.

Many gym memberships can be "frozen," which means that if you're not going for a month or two or ten you can pay a lower rate – a "freeze fee." It might be ten dollars instead of sixty. Joke and Waxworth started telling prospects that they'd get their first three months at a reduced rate (aka the freeze fee). This saved the member several hundred dollars – and cost the company the same. It was very easy to do, since the computer system couldn't retro-bill someone once they were taken off freeze.

The two of them were raking it in with this scam – and it was costing me plenty. They'd call up my prospects that were still on the fence and offer them their "deal," claiming they were the only ones authorized to give it. That last part was ingenious; it kept me from finding out and exposing them. And with me unable to match what they were offering (and not even knowing about it), my people kept signing up with them behind my back.

Eventually, one of my clients felt bad about it and told me what happened. I did some research and found out that over a half-dozen people had taken part in the con, and that was just over the last few weeks. I was furious and went to my manager. He made sure I got back partial commission for my lost sales and gave the two responsible a gentle slap on the wrist, but that was it – no write ups or reports to corporate.

The fly in the ointment for these two finally came when the company started running quarterly full-system scans. Their reports showed that Joke had used the freeze scam on more than forty members. When confronted, he vehemently denied everything, but it was all done from his computer, during his shift, and using his password.

After Joke was canned, and his members were forced to pay regular dues, the manager found a silver lining. Since he didn't want to lose *both* his sneaky salesmen, he used Joke's demise as an example to start making Waxworth do the right thing. Fear stopped his illegal activities dead in their tracks. But sadly, once he could no longer lie, cheat, and steal, his numbers were never the same.

SURVIVAL TIP #7

Be wary of gym deals that seem too good to be true. Especially if the sales rep seems ready to do anything to get you to sign, and if he's the kind of character you'd expect to come out of a dark alley with an armful of stolen watches.

If you do join based on some unusual arrangement, make damn sure any deal you've offered is documented in black and white, either on your contract or spelled out on company paperwork. Either way, try to get the manager to sign off on it – especially if parts seem questionable.

Many salespeople will say or do anything to get you to join. However, once you've signed and they've gotten paid, anything extraneous that they may have offered you will, most likely, never materialize.

If you do get conned and try to complain, your sales rep will undoubtedly develop selective memory loss. It'll be your word against theirs. So make sure you get everything in writing, and get that manager's signature! If you do, even if he or she no longer works there, the company will have no choice but to honor it.

CHARACTER SPOTLIGHT: THE KING

Without a doubt, my favorite gym con man was a sales associate at Empirical Sports who worked at one of our sister locations. He was a former city employee who, of all things, left the job to come and work in fitness. Let's call him "King."

King's manager made the mistake of giving him and another salesperson the authorized log-in codes. Presumably the manager did this to reduce his workload – so the two could make necessary commission adjustments on their sales when he wasn't available to do so. Obviously, he really trusted them.

You can do a lot with those codes.

Out of "nowhere," the two salespeople in question started getting unheard-of commissions. All their sales went up and up. Instead of getting say, $60 per sale, they were getting $90 or even $150. Over the next few months, they each raked in $16,000 dollars of extra cabbage. Things finally came to an end when whoever was making these illegal adjustments got lazy. Instead of putting in an extra $30 or $60 per sale (which wouldn't stand out much), they put in $1,000 instead! I guess it was an attempt to get more by doing less.

The glassy-eyed bean counters at payroll had failed to detect all the previous action, but this was something nobody could miss.

The manager was fired at once, as were the two salespeople. The company tried to press charges, but everyone denied any wrongdoing and blamed each other. Everything was theory and speculation, and no one would testify or offer any proof. Corporate tried hard to get even, or at least get their money back. They even attempted to coerce the two young people's parents into repaying the cash they'd "allegedly" taken.

Their calls were met with a resounding, "Go to hell."

It's no wonder that members' dues keep going up. Let's face it: *someone's* got to pay for all that missing money . . .

UNORTHODOX SELLING

Most salespeople get jaded after working in fitness for a while. They might grow weary making the same pitch thing day after day, hearing the same objections and excuses. Or perhaps they start looking down their noses at out-of-shape potential clients. Regardless of the reason, over the years I've seen gym salespeople become downright abusive.

And when that happens, *anything* is possible.

Before I went into sales at Caveat Sports, I witnessed my manager Robert abusing a blind man. As I passed his office, I noticed all the other sales reps and one of the receptionists gathered outside, laughing it up like they were at a comedy club. I drew closer, and observed Robert explaining rates to an elderly gentleman wearing dark glasses. At first, Robert seemed completely professional. But every once in a while, his facial expression became borderline diabolical. Out of nowhere, he'd thrust his hand in front of his visually-impaired client like a boxer's jab, giving him the bird from less than four inches away.

He did this repeatedly. And his staff loved it.

Eventually, the bewildered man started yelling, "Why's everyone laughing? Why do they keep laughing?"

When I worked at Empirical Sports, I witnessed a similar incident. One of my colleagues was in a foul mood. He'd been repeatedly trying to close a young, heavyset girl, but she kept wriggling out of his clutches. Exasperation finally set in. I heard him belt out, "You know you're fat, right? You know you need the gym, right?"

Things got a little less cordial after that.

Obviously, she didn't sign, but it didn't stop other people from trying similar closes.

I had a manager at Caveat Sports we'll call "Brass." He had plenty of it. One afternoon, he was trying to nail down what he called a "well-nourished" business woman. She was a tough cookie, and also a trifle rude. Suddenly, I heard the sales banter turn ugly. As she stood up to leave, Brass looked her up and down and said, "Lady, you're fat! Fat! If you don't join, your husband's gonna cheat on you and you're gonna have a heart attack and die!"

The poor woman burst into tears and ran out hysterical. Her husband called up ranting and raving. Brass told him – and this is a direct quote – "Yeah, that's right. I told your wife she's fat, and she *is*! And you know it too; you just don't have the balls to say it . . . You wanna do something about it? C'mon down. I'll kick your ass *and* your fat wife's!"

I'm not usually like that, but something similar happened when I was the manager of that same location. Three housewives came in at lunchtime and joined on impulse. While I was doing their paperwork (they were standing over me because they were in a rush), I made polite conversation, asking what kind of workouts they wanted to do (gain, lose, tone, etc.). One of them threw open her coat and struck a pose to show off her figure. "Do I look like I need to lose weight?" she asked.

When I made the mistake of following her display with my eyes, she snapped, "Are you checking me out?"

I shook my head and finished their paperwork, post haste.

Later that evening, the same woman called me and told me she and her friends changed their minds and wanted to cancel. I reiterated my company's money-back-guarantee policy. When she discovered she couldn't kill her membership off over the phone she grew hostile. An hour later, her husband called me and accused me of misleading my clients and then started threatening me. "You deceive people when they join, and I'm going to make sure you don't get away with it anymore."

I wasn't in the mood for any abuse. I told him to take his best shot. Then I added (as *professionally* as possible) that, if he felt the need to express himself further, I'd be happy to discuss the matter face to face. I let him know what time I got off to make sure he wouldn't miss me.

Sorry to say, he never showed up.

That was too damned bad. Not to sound like a thug, but my knees were really aching that day. I would have enjoyed resting them on his chest for a while.

SURVIVAL TIP #8

Unless you're an MMA contender looking for some impromptu action, mouthing off to a health club employee – especially a trainer or manager – is hazardous to one's health. Besides their above-average supply of muscle, a lot of people in the fitness industry have extensive training in mixed-martial arts and boxing. Some also have backgrounds in security-related fields, such as personal protection or nightclub work.

That being said – look before leaping.

CHAPTER 6:

THE SELLING PROCESS,
PART 1: OPENING SALVOS

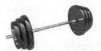

Three things happen when someone considers joining a health club: the *Info calls*, the *Greeting*, and the *Needs Analysis*. I've provided a brief description of each, followed by detailed breakdowns so you know exactly what's going on when you experience them.

- *Info calls* take place when a client picks up the phone and calls a club. Usually, the caller is interested in getting price information. The person they speak to will have something entirely different in mind.
- The *Greeting* takes place when a potential client walks into a health club. The salesperson will approach and address you in a fairly predictable manner. Watch out for the *way* you're greeted; it can often tell you the temperament and proficiency of the rep you're dealing with.
- Last but not least, the *Needs Analysis* is an informal interview wherein a client sits down with their prospective salesperson, typically prior to taking a tour. It may appear to be a Q&A session, with the sales rep kindly helping you to achieve your goals. What's really happening is far more insidious.

INFO CALLS

Phone inquiries are the lifeblood of salespeople the world over – in gyms even more so. The goal, naturally, is to have the caller make an appointment, and then come in and join (and hopefully bring their friends). From the salesperson's POV, info calls are invaluable, as they lead to additional sales beyond street traffic and referrals.

The moment you ask for membership information, you become a target. The receptionist may sound all sweetness and light, but the moment they put you on hold, you cease to be a human being. They'll page the next available sales rep, informing them, "Attention "Joe," info call on line two."

Editor's Note: Don't be surprised if the receptionist also asks for your phone number. Usually this is done "in case you get disconnected." Phone systems are hardly so shoddy. They're trained to get your number in advance, so that if the sales rep fails to get an appointment out of you, they can follow up until they manage to do so. Be wary of giving out your number.

When it comes to distributing info calls, different places have different policies. For example, Caveat Sports allows the manager to control everything; thus, they have the power to give walk-ins and info calls to whosoever they see fit. Or they can keep everything for themselves . . .

Dinar Fitness was more interesting. They had a "jungle rules" system. When a phone inquiry came in, the front desk girl simply announced it – *"Attention team, info call on line one!"*

Then follows a mad stampede for the phones; people will literally run over each other, pushing, shoving, and elbowing to be the first to get the call. Fights and scuffles were common. You had to be fast on your feet and able to take a few shots if you wanted to get one of those calls.

Of course, weasel that I'd become, and too lazy to make the dash, I came up with a cunning technique that netted me nearly all the calls. I simply stayed in my office. As soon as I heard an announcement that started with: *"Attention team—"* I jabbed that blinking line faster than Muhammad Ali in his prime. Two out of three times, it was something worthless, like a personal call for a colleague or a member rescheduling with their trainer. When that happened, I just smiled through the phone and replied: "Sure, no problem. Let me get him for you."

But every so often, my aggressiveness was rewarded with those delightful words that sent shivers down my spine, all the way to my wallet.

"Hi, how much is it to join?"

My lips spread into a grin, followed by my usual, "Sure, thing. I'm Max, What's your name?"

I'd be reticent in my duties if I didn't touch on phone scripts. Sales reps are trained not only on how to answer the phone, but also how to control the conversation. Reps try to avoid giving you prices over the phone. If the rates are unattractive, they can't stop you from hanging up. They'd prefer to keep you in their office as a figurative prisoner. If their gym is as pricey as some of the places I've worked, they need to do that in order to justify the price and manipulate you mentally.

A typical info call starts with the company's standard greeting: "Caveat Sports, this is Max." Sales reps are trained to smile when they talk and to control their voice inflections over the phone, so don't be surprised when they sound genuinely friendly.

A potential client usually responds to this greeting with either: "How much is it to join?" or "Hi, I'm interested in signing up." Either way, the rep attempts to subtly seize control of the conversation. This varies from person to person, but my technique was to sound agreeable: "Sure, I'm Max. And you are?"

This forces the caller to give their name – an elicited, instinctive response. Before the caller can regroup the rep starts to steer. "Hi, 'Jake,' what can I do for you?" It sounds harmless enough, but when the caller starts pushing for prices ("How much are your memberships?") the salesperson remains unruffled and flows into, "Sure, Jake. Is it for you or you and a friend?"

Some people assume the rep is trying to get an extra sale – and they'll certainly take one if it's offered – but this is more of a distraction. Regardless of the answer, the next question is typically, "Great. What are you looking to do in terms of a workout?"

The rep couldn't care less what the client is looking to accomplish. Again, this is a misdirection technique to keep them off balance and not focusing on what they called for. It's all smoke and mirrors.

Sooner or later, the sale rep tries to set up an appointment for the caller. "That sounds terrific, Jake. We can definitely do that for you. When do you want to come down? I have appointments available this afternoon or this evening. Which works best for you?"

Notice the ongoing agreeability and how words like "Sure" and "Great" are thrown in to make it seem like the caller has their rep's support and approval and that they're in charge. They're not. Also, notice the "either or" closing technique. I didn't ask *if* the caller wanted to come down. I'm *assuming* they do. It's hard to resist a question like that.

If the caller is really adamant about getting prices, the dance will continue. If someone was really stubborn, I'd note that they hadn't seen the gym yet. "Look, I appreciate where you're coming from, but the company doesn't let me give prices over the phone – especially to someone that hasn't even seen the club." Then, I'd add, "They want you to come down and see what you're getting for your money, so you know you're going to be happy. I think it's a smart move. You wouldn't buy a car without at least seeing it and test driving it, right?"

What's the caller going to say at that point?

If need be, I'd tout the great facility I had to offer, topped off with a list of amenities (specifically tailored to their goals, which they already gave me) that made clients feel like they were joining a five-star spa. I'd promise them that the price was so great for what they were getting, it'd blow their minds – and that I personally guaranteed to not pressure them.

Sooner or later, they'd weary of the chess match and cave. I was very good when it came to info calls; my call-to-appointment ratio was nearly 90%

In the innuendo-laced words of my Regional Director, I "gave good phone."

PHONE WARS

When money is involved, things always have the potential to go awry. And since every info call is a potential sale (or two), people will try to steal them.

When I worked at Empirical Sports, our front desk monitored the info calls. They kept track of everything by using an "up system." This system was designed to level the playing field and make sure everyone took turns. The concept worked well, unless the receptionist had a crush on one of the salespeople (an enviable situation I found myself in more than once). Like any system, however, there were ways to milk it.

One day, I found myself working with what I'll politely call a pair of less-than-upstanding individuals. Their names were "Panini" and "Antoine," and they were as sneaky and underhanded as salespeople come. Yet as treacherous as they were, they had a hard time hitting the numbers. They decided to try a unique approach at stealing info calls. They'd check the up-sheet and wait until I was next in queue. Then, they'd have one of their friends call from their house, pretending to be interested in membership. This third party would then make a fake appointment, allowing either Panini or Antoine the opportunity to steal the next real call.

The tactic worked a few times, but fortunately I catch on quick. The co-conspirators made stupid mistakes, like acquiescing to an appointment too easily, or boasting that they had two or more friends coming with them, all of whom were "definitely joining." Things like that don't happen often. When they failed to show and their numbers turned out to be bogus, I figured out what was going on.

My solution was simple (*no*, it didn't involved dragging one of them outside by the nape and beating the snot out of him). The next time an "info call" was transferred to me, I made the appointment, and then called back immediately.

Disconnected.

I immediately got up and told the receptionist to uncheck me – that the call wasn't a true info call, just an active member asking for info on an existing contract. And I made sure my "colleague" Panini in the next office overheard this. Predictably, he tried to make an issue out of it.

"That was an info call!" he exclaimed.

I gave him a curious look. "No, it *wasn't*," I said. "And how would you know? Were *you* on the phone? No. So mind your business."

After having dealt with this situation and others, I developed a simple technique for making sure info calls were legit. I called it "de-fanging the serpent." It was a practical necessity. Even if I wasn't working with borderline criminals, I'd get a lot of fake calls anyway. They might be from bored clients looking to jerk my chain, other clubs harassing the competition, or even my own corporate office checking up on my phone technique – there was always something.

My new method was flawless. When someone asked for pricing I'd say, "Sure, I'm Max. And you are?" Once they introduced themselves I'd quickly interject, "Listen, 'Joe,' I'd *love* to help you, but I'm by myself here and in the middle of doing memberships for these guys (the "guys" were fictitious, of course). Do you have a number I can call you back at?"

If necessary, I'd even improvise a quick conversation with my invisible "new members" to illustrate their impatience: "Just one second guys . . . I'm so sorry." This not only made it more believable, but if the caller was genuine, it whetted their appetite to get in on my "big sale."

And *nobody* wants to miss a sale.

It separated the wheat from the chaff. You could sense a fake caller's immediate annoyance when they realized they'd been neutralized. They'd cop an attitude, decline giving their number, and say they'd call back (never happened). If it was the office calling, they thought I was setting the world on fire, and serious parties *gladly* gave me their number. Not only were they definitely legit, but I had their number – a vital indication of their interest.

THE GREETING

When you're learning to sell gym memberships, one of the first things they drill into your head is how to greet potential clients at the front desk. You're supposed to be cheery and appreciative of this rare and wonderful person who has graciously come for you to enlighten them about the gift of fitness.

For the record, that's balderdash. Salespeople are conditioned to act that way (regardless of their actual mood), and while doing so, they're envisioning a big pile of dollar bills where that person is standing. The more talented reps are so smooth you'd be amazed. They'll beam at you, shake your hand, and look you in the eye with complete sincerity. They're like bloodsucking vampires, preparing to hypnotize their next victim.

Remember, it's all about the money. A prospect walking into the club is never referred to by name, at least not amongst the staff. They're not "Jane" or "John" (although they should be). They're either a "walk-in" or an "up." That means they either walked in without an appointment, or they're to be handed to the next person on the up system.

Editor's Note: Walk-ins are eminently desirable. They're much more likely to join than the guest of an existing member. Guests are usually just there to keep their friend company. Walk-ins usually come in because they're actually interested in joining.

CHARACTER SPOTLIGHT: TONGUE TIED

Sometimes sales reps get bored with the pretense and start looking for new and creative ways to do things, even something as simple as saying hello. My old manager Robert was a perfect example. He'd stand behind the front desk and mutter perverse things under his breath that most people wouldn't catch. And if they did, he'd make sure he had a back-up ready – some harmless phrase that was similar enough to pull it off.

Once, I watched an elderly Russian woman walk in. She pointed past the front desk, to a glass door overlooking the aerobics studio. There was a class going on, and she pointed and asked in broken English, "My . . . friend. I . . . look?"

Robert gave her a huge smile and said, "Sure, go right on back and press your nose up against my scrotum."

Her head bobbed up and down in agreement as she walked away.

I almost died.

As luck would have it, Robert got himself in trouble more than once with these romper room antics. One day, a middle-aged, bottom-heavy woman came in and scanned her card. He must have assumed she was Russian, because he looked at her, nodded, and said with a smile, "Shaped like a bell."

Unfortunately for him, the woman was Italian, and a native New Yorker. She gave him a withering stare and repeated angrily, *"Shaped like a bell?"*

My eyes bugged out. I could hear Robert panic as he stammered, "No, no . . . I said I can *tell*. You've lost weight, I can *tell*!"

I walked away to avoid being seen laughing. Meanwhile, the woman sized Robert up with a look that suggested she would drag him outside, wedge him under the wheel well of a car, and stomp him half to death.

He chose his victims more carefully after that.

THE HIGHEST FORM OF FLATTERY

Young and impressionable pup that I was, I inevitably picked up some of Robert's bad habits. One time, a family of four was waiting for me in the lobby. I had a small chalk board in my office that I used to leave reminders for myself. I grabbed some chalk powder and smeared it on and under my nose, then came bursting out of my office like a maniac, eyes wild and chest heaving. I charged up to them, fists clenched, and bellowed, "Alright! Who wants to work out? Let's *do this*!!!"

The family's eyes flew open wide in collective horror. They fell back over one another, trampling the smaller members of their group as they scrambled out the door and ran for their lives.

As funny as it was, I regretted the gag. It cost me over a hundred dollars, just to have a laugh.

Some days, if I was bored, I'd walk around and greet existing members, which could be almost as much fun. You'd be surprised by the looks you get when you walk up to a pulchritudinous female with a bag of Planters in your hand and ask "Would you like some penis?"

Obviously, after her look of outrageous indignation ("What the *hell* did you just say?"), it was a simple matter to innocently reply, "I said, would you like some *peanuts*," while holding up the proffered gift.

Worked every time.

My favorites were the ones where the member's name was just *begging* to be used.

I had a silver-haired client at Caveat Sports named *Semen* (in Russian it's Simon). I *loved* going up to gym floor at rush hour. I'd spot him from far off and yell at the top of my lungs, "Semen! Yo, Semen!" Clients and trainers stared, horror-stricken, at my crotch. Of course, poor Semen had no idea anything was amiss. He thought I was genuinely happy to see him, and smiled and waved back like everything was great. Which, naturally, made it all the better. Plausible deniability is a great thing.

Now that you've heard about my pal Semen, you don't even *want* to know about my other Russian client.

Her honest-to-God first name was *Vagina* . . .

NEEDS ANALYSIS

All salespeople are trained to go through what's known as the "Needs Analysis." This is the one you really want to be on your toes for. It's where the salesperson tries to get to know you – your interests and desires (aka your *needs*). In reality, they're just pinpointing your weaknesses. They've been trained to pick you apart and find out what they need to say.

What must they do for you to give them your money? It's more than just giving you a good deal. Are you a skinny teen who's been picked on and wants to be big and strong and able to fight back? Are you a horny guy who wants six-pack abs so you can go to the beach and land more girls? Or are you a distraught housewife who discovered your husband is banging your younger sister because you never lost that baby weight, and now you want to get revenge by looking amazing?

Be aware of the questions you're asked and the answers you give. Remember, anything you say can and will be used against you.

Over the years I've heard all the stories. I interviewed one guy at Caveat Sports who told me point blank, "Look, Max. Let me be honest with you. I got absolutely no interest whatsoever in working out. I'm here for pussy, pure and simple. You okay with that?"

Wow. Even if I wasn't, I still would have said "yes." For sure, I didn't realize how serious this pervert actually was. A few days later, he walked into the aerobics studio in the middle of an abs class. There were twenty-five women there, lying on their backs, with their legs spread wide as they did crunches. He weaved his way in and around them like he was shopping the supermarket meat counter, grinning as he unabashedly ogled their crotches.

Needless to say, I had to have a conversation with him after that. It wasn't a red light district, after all.

A client at Empirical Sports named "Joseph" came to me distraught. "Max, I got a treadmill in my house that cost five thousand bucks. I can't use it. I'm on it not for five minutes before my wife starts yelling and screaming about how she needs a check for this, cash for that . . . I can't get a moment's peace. I can't take it!"

"So, what I can I do for you?" I asked.

"Simple, you let me pay for this anyway I want, right?"

"Sure. What did you have in mind?"

Joseph pulled out his wallet. "I'm using my business credit card and corporate address for the account. That way she knows nothing. You want a phone number? I got a cell phone she don't know about, too."

I shrugged. "Whatever you need, Joe. It's fine by me."

He smiled and handed me his card. "This place is my *sanctuary*, Max. When I'm here, she don't know where I am and she can't bother me. I come here, I get some peace."

I absolutely *loved* this guy. He was as direct as they come. And he wasn't kidding. Every day I'd see him walk in and stop outside my office. He'd raise his arms out to the side and suck in a huge breath, like he'd just gotten out of prison. Then he'd give a huge smile and run into the gym like it was the gates of Elysium.

This went on for months. One day, Joe disappeared. I don't know if he started going to a different location, or if his wife tracked him down and castrated him. I was afraid to call. I can definitely say, though, that my club made a *huge* difference in his life; he was by far the most henpecked client I ever had.

I miss that guy.

NEEDS ANALYSIS GONE WRONG

Once in a while, I'd sit down with potential customers who were so uptight I had to do crazy things to break the ice. Whether it was cracking self-deprecating jokes, or licking my fingertip and then tickling one of my nipples (yes, one must establish a *certain* degree of comfort before doing so), I did whatever needed to be done.

If the need arose, I could do a number of animal sound effects, including an ultra-realistic pig impersonation for some guys (as an obese girl passed outside my office) that had them peeing in their pants. If it helped make people laugh, I did an assortment of comedic foreign accents: Indian, Scottish, Russian, Italian . . . you name it. One time, this Irish woman at U.S. Amazing Fitness got annoyed at me trying to bond with her. She told me, "You Americans think you're pretty funny with your little leprechaun accents. But we Irish don't talk like that, we talk like *this*. And if ya don't cut it out I'm gonna hit ya in the head!"

Since I wasn't in the mood to get beat up by a woman (at least, not without having paid for it), I acquiesced to her desires.

My favorite client interviews, however, were with people who could have been escapees from a popular TV show. I had one customer, a beautiful Egyptian woman, who was perfect in every way except one: her hands were like calloused catcher's mitts. No joke; she had paws like a concrete statue. It took a lot of willpower for me to ignore her mannish meat hooks and focus on what she was saying. Unfortunately, one of the trainers at Empirical Sports wasn't so compassionate. He made a snide comment she caught wind of and she canceled her membership a day later.

So much for *that* commission.

Another time I had a "low-talker" who spoke in such hushed tones I thought I was going deaf. We're talking whispers. I had to lean so far over my desk I nearly fell into her lap. It was beyond difficult, trying to pre-close a sale when every other word out of my mouth was, "What was that?"

The absolute crème de la crème though, was an honest-to-God "close-talker." I didn't think people like this actually existed, but I was wrong. I was called to the front, where a tall, well-dressed gentleman was waiting. As I shook his hand, he took a big step forward, moving so close to me it was unsettling. The guy was two inches away. I actually thought he was going to kiss me.

I took a quick step back, but this particular close-talker anticipated my reaction and moved with me like it was a choreographed dance. It was like we were crazy-glued together. I turned my head to the side so he wouldn't see me crack up. The only word I managed was, "*Dude!*" before I started chuckling.

When the guy realized that he couldn't stay face to face with me, he settled for moving next to me. He followed me throughout the club, hip to hip. In my office, he leaned so far over the desk, I felt like *I* was a low-talker. I felt bad for him; he must have suffered a terrible case of separation anxiety during childhood that made him that way.

Whatever it was, the guy definitely had much ado about *something* going on.

SURVIVAL TIP #9

All jokes aside, when contacting a health club about membership, keep your wits about you. And be prepared to jump some hurdles

Don't give out your phone number unless you feel comfortable. You can say you're calling from work, that you're using a borrowed cell phone, or that you just flat out don't give away your private number. It's up to you. The last thing you want, should you decide you're not interested, is to get pushy sales calls every day for six months. It happens all the time.

If you find yourself in a gym, remember, that charming sales- man who's schmoozing you is just looking to make a commis- sion. A week after you've joined, he probably won't recognize you. Sales reps deal with thousands of members; it's impossible to remember them all, no matter how good you are. A client once criticized me by telling my boss that when I signed him up, I acted like his best friend. He said it felt like I just pulled him out of a smoking foxhole. A few days later, however, I couldn't recall his name. In my defense, I wasn't trying to be phony with the guy. But when you've signed up over 20,000 people, your brain can only handle so much.

Last, but not least, be extra alert during your interview. The sales rep will ask you things like how long it's been since you exercised, if you have the support of friends and family, or how long it's been since you were happy with the way you look. These questions are not there to make you feel better by open- ing up. You're not talking to a shrink. You're talking to a seller of goods. Their questions are designed to give them ammuni- tion to use against you. They expose the chinks in your psycho- logical armor, and they will exploit those vulnerabilities later, should you hesitate to sign up after your tour.

There's nothing worse than hearing, "But Jane, you just told me fifteen minutes ago that you've been miserable with your body since you got pregnant, that your husband hardly touches you anymore, and that you want to feel attractive again. You've waited five years to take this step. Why talk yourself out of it now?"

Remember, think like a fighter: always keep your guard up.

CHAPTER 7:

THE SELLING PROCESS, PART 2: SURVIVING THE BATTLE

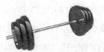

I've already covered the greeting and the interview process. Now, I'm going to delve into what takes place during your tour of the actual facility and the price presentation that will follow.

THE TOUR

When I was in sales, my favorite part of membership presentations was the tour. Some of my employers didn't feel tours were important, some recommended avoiding them altogether, but I relished them. It gave me the chance to use my personality to get potential clients to relax so I could bond with them.

In the fitness industry the "powers that be" like to think of the whole meet-and-greet/tour/pricing routine as an inverted pyramid. They feel that most of a sales rep's time should be spent doing the needs analysis and less doing tours. By the time they've brought their prospect back to the office for price presentation and close, the prospect should already be 90% sold.

There is some truth to this. If you're going to be in a gunfight, you should load your weapon before the shooting starts. A salesman will try to get to know you, inside out and backwards, before they try to sell you. They may forget you even *exist* an hour or two after you join, but until then, they'll seem so close you'll feel like they just pulled you out of a burning car wreck.

Starting during your needs analysis and continuing into your tour, your salesperson will ask you what are known as "leading questions," designed to feel you out and subtly put you in a buying mindset. You'll hear things like: "How many days per week are you planning to work out?" and, "How long has it been since you worked out regularly? Why did you stop? What's different now that makes you feel you're going to stick with it?" Then there's: "Do you have your spouse's/family's support?"

Does any of this sound familiar?

It should if you've ever joined a gym. These questions make you start to commit subconsciously, long before price negotiations start. And, they give your sales rep ammo to use against you later. Like when you start voicing what are referred to as "objections" (we'll discuss those when we get to "The Close").

A lot of sales reps also do what are known as "trial closes" during a tour. It's a very sneaky technique – one that even a savvy customer often fails to pick up on because they're distracted by all the equipment and amenities. The rep will ask things like: "So, will you be doing most of your training up here with the cardio equipment, or do you plan on hitting the weights more?" Another sequence might be, "Do you want to see the locker room? Will you be using the showers? If you're going to, we also offer complimentary towel service."

An experienced salesperson can tell whether or not you're likely to join based on how you answer these questions. I always could. I eventually wouldn't even bother with such tactics unless I suspected someone was wasting my time. In that case, trial closes were a good way to find out if it was worth expending any energy on them.

Only fight the fights you can win.

One technique is called "personalizing the tour" – going beyond just showing clients the equipment. I would put the tour into the "possessive tense." I wanted prospects to feel like they owned the gym, that it was already theirs. I'd say things like: "Here's the free weights you wanted, Bob. This is where you're going to build those guns you want, big guy." And for women: "Jane, this is *your* aerobic studio, where you're going to get those flat, toned abs you were talking about. This is *your* locker room, Sara, where you can shower before going back to work. This is *your* steam and sauna . . ."

And so forth.

SMOKE AND MIRRORS

I've told you about tours. One point I haven't touched on, however, is that many clubs actually *skip* the tour portion of their pitch. Caveat Sports was notorious for this. I remember a sales training class, hosted by our notorious

Regional Director, Jack Daniels. He told us point blank: *"Why take people on a tour of your club? Don't do that. What if it's dirty or crowded or smelly? What if no one from management ever sets foot on the gym floor, and all of a sudden, there you are? Why risk getting swarmed by complaining members, bitching and moaning about crowded conditions, broken machines, or what-not? Why risk losing the sale? Don't give tours, just take them in an office and beat them over the head until they join!"*

Surprisingly, this tactic is fairly common, especially in clubs that shirk their housekeeping and maintenance duties. When I worked for Caveat Sports, I was forced to use it as a survival tool. Of course, if people *wanted* to see the place I smiled and grudgingly showed them around, but this was like playing Russian roulette. *"Is the place clean? Is my client able to see the bottom of the pool? Are guys masturbating in the steam room?"*

Just a few of the worries I carried around.

Fortunately, most places I worked were presentable enough to help close sales. Empirical Sports was except for the men's locker room, a perpetual pig sty that I avoided like the plague. It was strewn with trash and dirty towels, not to mention toilets clogged and filled to overflowing with what I'll politely refer to as Lincoln logs.

Would *you* pay $75 a month for that?

Selling is hard enough already. Still, one must rise to overcome such obstacles. I adopted a technique many women use to get rid of a guy: I avoided them. If I knew the locker room was a shambles and a client asked to see it, I tried screwing with their heads to change their minds. It was easy – I'd play on their instinctive fears. Most men, when told, "it's your basic locker room – steam room, sauna – and a lot of naked men walking around . . ." will quickly lose interest. Especially if you ask them in front of their friends, *"Do you want to see some naked guys?"*

What's the guy going to say? *"Wow, a sausage-fest? Sure, count me in!"*

Homophobia: it is a many-splendored thing.

On days when touring the locker room was unavoidable, I fell back on my most reliable asset – my sense of humor. No matter what, I always tried to have my clients laughing their asses off while I showed them around. This made closing the sale more likely, plus they'd be distracted from noticing potential problems (leaking ceilings, defective water fountains, a dozen machines with "Out of Order" signs. . .). I told the same jokes on every tour, but it didn't matter to new customers – they were seeing the show for the first time.

"Here's the aerobics studio, guys. This is where we keep all the appetizers – I mean entrees – I mean group exercise equipment!"

"Girls, this is the ladies locker room. I'm not allowed in there anymore ever since 'the incident,' so if you don't mind, I'll wait out here . . ."

"Here's your gym floor, brother. There's enough iron down here to build a battleship, and when we're done, your guns will be just as big!"

"Is the Jacuzzi clean? Oh, definitely; we change the water daily. Personally, I don't relish basting myself in some old guy's ball juice . . . but hey, if that's what you're into, it's fine by me!"

After watching me compliment a particularly hairy (and shirtless) client on his "sweater," or seeing me pause on the gym floor to tell a member (who looked remarkably like Richard Attenborough), *"I loved you in Jurassic Park,"* prospects were so entertained they wouldn't notice if the place was on fire.

My clients were awesome.

CHARACTER SPOTLIGHT: TOUR DE FARCE

There is a certain breed of individual who likes to tour health clubs with absolutely no interest in joining. They'll go to a gym, sit through the whole needs analysis, do the tour, and then announce that they're not looking to join.

Why they do this, I have absolutely no idea, but it is aggravating for those of us with bills to pay. It wastes the salesperson's time and energy. And it's a major tease and let-down.

One time, I took this guy "Fred" on a tour. We bonded for a good twenty minutes in the office before going on to see the club. Then, when the price sheets came out, he told me, "Oh, I'm not looking to join."

"You're not?" I asked, confused. "Well, you certainly seemed inclined to when we discussed you losing twenty pounds and getting your energy levels back."

"Yeah, but that was just because I wanted to see the place."

"Excuse me?"

He nodded. "I just wanted to check out the club. You know . . . see what it was all about."

This annoyed me. "Are you telling me you came all the way here and spent forty minutes with me, but you never had any intention of signing up?"

"Yeah. Why, is that bad?"

I don't remember if I was having a bad day prior to that or not, but this had steam coming out of my ears.

"Is there something wrong with you?" I asked. "Are you some kind of sick fuck who likes to go to gyms and waste salespeople's time? Seriously, do you get some twisted pleasure from jerking people around making them *think* you're going to join, when you have no interest whatsoever?"

Paling in the face of my self-righteous indignation, Fred tried to stutter a mealy mouthed apology, but I cut him off. I stood up, opened my office door, and told him, "Get out, and don't ever come back."

There've been a few incidents like that. One guy waded through the tour and pricing, then smiled smugly and leaned back in his chair. He folded his arms across his chest and told me, "I'm not ready to join right now. I'm going to have to *think* about it."

Unfortunately for Mister TIO (Think It Over) I had a couple of b-backs (people I'd already seen that came back to join) smiling and waving at me as they waited outside my office. Frankly, I didn't like TIO's smirking demeanor, and being one to always go with the proverbial "bird in the hand," I stood up, shook his hand while simultaneously grabbing his forearm and elbow, and hoisted him to his feet.

I smirked back at him. "You're absolutely right. This is a big decision. You *should* go home and think about it. Give me call when you've made up your mind." Without another word I ushered him out the door and waved my waiting couple in. They nodded amiably at him as they passed by, credit cards in hand, and I never gave him another glance. He stood there flabbergasted, staring forlornly through the glass for a good thirty seconds before he finally walked out.

As one of my co-workers used to say, "Guaranteed sales are like loose women; always go with a sure thing."

The funniest part of that little encounter was that after he'd gotten over the initial shock, TIO was so irate that he *had* to join. I suppose he wasn't good at handling rejection. He came back to the club when I wasn't there and joined with another rep, but requested I not receive credit for the sale because he "didn't like me."

Of course, my co-worker and I had a good working relationship, so he told me about it, and I *did* get the credit.

THE CLOSE

The absolute climax of any sales presentation is what's known as "the close." It's when the salesperson aggressively tries to seal the deal – to overcome your objections (your reasons for saying "no") and get you to say "yes" – in this case, to a gym membership.

The close is the most stressful portion of the selling process, by far. It's the endgame – the final decision. The pressure is on for both of you. It's predator vs. prey – good deal for you vs. a big commission for them.

But will you join, or won't you?

The subchapters below show you what to expect so you're better prepared to emerge victorious. And who knows? Just maybe, armed with the knowledge I'm giving you, *you'll* be the one to walk away licking your fangs.

Whatever the case, the watering hole will never be the same . . .

CLOSING COSTS

Over the course of my years in sales, I learned numerous closing techniques, ranging from the basic "A or B" close (silver or gold?), to the more advanced and complicated "reduction to the ridiculous" gambit (wherein you break your club's monthly dues or PIF price down to a daily dollar amount that appears so small, it's impossible to balk at).

For now, let's focus on the latter.

A Caveat Sports member walked into Empirical Sports one day because his three-year contract was over – a common occurrence. He told me he was fed up with the place and looking to jump ship. Let's call him "Abdul."

Abdul's main beef with Caveat Sports was the interminable wait for equipment, especially at peak hours. With their clubs statistically averaging 10,000-plus members apiece, at rush hour it was like exercising in an overheated sardine can.

It smelled like one too.

Abdul loved my facility, and we hit it off. When he found out that we had ten treadmills and six benches free even at our busiest times, he thought he'd entered the gates of Shangri La.

Everything seemed like a slam-dunk – until I told him the price. Suddenly, paying over seventy bucks a month for "paradise" was too much, especially compared to the twelve dollars a month he was shelling out for the other place.

Undaunted by Abdul's unexpected reticence, I smiled and went to work. Moments like that – when I realized a prospect wasn't going to be an easy kill – were when I "punched in." In other words, I'd quit playing around and unleash my full arsenal of sales skills.

Like I said previously, the industry had turned me into something not-so-nice.

I focused on Abdul's main complaint, his current club's overcrowded workout conditions. I asked him how many days a week he used his current club (it was five, God bless) and how long his average workout was (3.5 hours). Then I asked him how much time he spent waiting for machines (an hour and a half).

I grabbed my calculator and did some quick fingering. Based on Abdul's three-year contract, I deduced that Caveat Sports had basically stolen 1,170 hours of his *life*. That equated to forty eight *days*. And those were 24/7 days, not eight hour shifts. I told him that I had no idea how much he got paid at his job, but that he'd spent a month and a half of his life standing around his gym, "waiting with his thumb stuck up his butt" (his exact words), in the hopes of getting to use their "worn out machines" (again, his words). Could that sacrifice of time possibly compare to investing a mere $60 more per month – less than $15 per week – for him to have his freedom back?

Abdul pursed his lips. Then he threw his Visa card at me.

SALES SCRIPTS – I OBJECT!

Although the aforementioned sale ended amiably, that's the exception to the rule. Anyone checking out a gym must keep in mind that health clubs train their sales staff to close people aggressively, using tried-and-true formulas. As a result, potential members are usually treated to a "sales script," a prearranged series of prying questions and answers, designed to systematically herd them into buying.

The most successful (and formidable) sales reps skip using selling scripts altogether; in fact, they disdain them. Instead, they function instinctively, mentally and emotionally merging with their clients, subtly altering their mannerisms, speech patterns, and the tone of their voice, until they can bond with just about anyone, from politicians to pimps.

With the exception of these elite (known in the industry as "chameleons"), however, the majority of reps do rely on their scripts.

I've listed a few basic Q&As so you know what to watch for. Joining a gym should be *your* decision, based on satisfaction with product and price – not because someone played with your head.

- Question 1: *"How long have you been thinking about joining the gym/ working out/losing all that weight . . . a day or two?"*

This question is asked (and partially answered, if you noticed) because the rep wants to manipulate you into admitting some forethought. If you say three months or (even better) three years, it gives them a powerful tool to use later, should you hesitate.

Let's assume you *have* been procrastinating for three years. The rep will reinforce your words (again, to use against you later) by asking a leading question like, *"Wow, three years. Good for you. I'm proud of you. So you've fi-nally decided it's time, yes?"*

If you answer in the affirmative, you give them what they want. Later, if you say you need time to think, they will reply, *"But John, you already told me you've been waiting three years to lose that gut and get the six-pack you've al-ways dreamed of. You said you were ready, right? I'm here for you, so let's do this!"*

- Question 2: *"How long has it been since your body/weight/physique was the way you want it?"*
  Again, your reply will also be held against you. Say you tell them you were nineteen, and now you're forty. That gives your rep twenty one years of procrastination that they can use to guilt you into joining. But what the heck; better late than never.
- Question 3: *"How long has it been since you were a member of a gym? Why did you quit/stop? Is that still a problem for you?"*

The rep wants to know if you were a member somewhere else. Your an-swer will give them an idea how much experience you have dealing with their kind, as well as how much you were paying and the quality of service (or lack thereof) you were getting.

Once they discover it's been three years (for example), watch for ques-tions 1 and 2, because they're coming. Also, the rep is trying to find out why you quit because they want to discover your hidden objections. If you say, *"I left because I broke my leg,"* or *"I was working two jobs and had no time,"* I guaran-tee you'll hear, *"But your leg's okay now, yes?"* or *"But you have time now, right?"*

The last thing a salesperson wants is an injury or time issue getting in the way of their commission.

- Question 4: *"How many days per week/what days do you plan on coming?"*

This is what's known as a "trial close": an attempt to get you to uncon-sciously commit. If you say you're coming three days per week, you've not only shown you're serious about joining, you've made a mental commitment. Your best bet when responding to this question would be, *"I'm not sure yet."*

Salespeople *hate* non-committal responses like that.

- Question 5: *"Is there anything you're looking for you haven't seen?"*

This question is designed to show you the club can provide you with everything you want. If there's anything they *don't* have, your rep will want to know ahead of time, so they can prepare a response.

- Question 6: *"Is your husband/wife/girlfriend/boyfriend excited about you joining the gym/losing weight/looking great?"*

This one's obvious. They want to remove one of the most annoying objections – the spousal. *"I don't know; I have to ask my (significant other) before I can sign up."* If you already told them your wife/husband is fired up about you joining you can't use them as an excuse. Also, if you *don't* have a significant other, keep quiet. Your best response? *"I don't know. We haven't discussed it yet."*

Editor's Note: at this point, a really pushy salesperson will have the nerve to tell you to call your significant then and there, so they can "help" you make a decision. This is greedy and grasping, but it happens all the time.

- Question 7: *"Okay, so based on what you told me your needs are, it sounds like our silver package works best for you, right?"*

This is designed to narrow down your choices. On the surface it looks like they want to pick out the best package for you, but in reality they're trying to paint you into a corner and cut off your escape routes. They want you to say "yes," because by doing so you're agreeing with them, and hence, selling yourself. Doesn't that make sense?

See, you just agreed with *me*!

Your best response to this would be, *"Maybe, but I want to take my time and consider my options."* By saying this, you tell them you're not ready to join yet and aren't to be rushed.

- Question 8: *"Is it in your budget/affordable for you?"*

This is pretty direct stuff. The rep wants to take price objection off the table. Once you say it's in your budget, you can't pull a 180 and say you can't afford it. A simple, *"I'm not sure,"* or *"I'll have to check,"* will do the job.

- Question 9: *"Isn't that a great deal for what you're getting?"*

Similar to the preceding question – they often accompany one another. Remember, just because something's a great deal doesn't mean it's in your budget.

- Question 10: *"How much would you be willing to spend per day to lose all that weight and keep it off? Five dollars . . . ten dollars?"*

Questions like this one are great; I've used them myself. If someone states how much they're willing to spend to achieve their goals, the rep has gotten a bit of financial commitment from them. Ten bucks a day sounds cheap, right? In a few minutes, when you find out the gym costs $75.00 per month and balk, your rep will say to you: *"But John, you just told me you're willing to spend ten dollars a day to lose that gut and feel great. That'd be $300.00 a month. We're charging you less than a quarter of that. Isn't that amazing?"*

For the record, if it was *me*, I'd really go for the kill. I'd hit you with: *"John, you just said you're willing to pay $300 a month, right? I'm charging you a fraction of that – more like $2.00 a day – plus I'm throwing in a $90 personal training session to get you started, and giving you a seven-day money-back guarantee on top of it. Try it for a week; if you're not happy you pay nothing. And the session – with that hot lady trainer you were checking out – is on me! You can't go wrong. The only thing you have to lose is pounds and inches. Am I right? Of course I am! What's it gonna be, gold or silver? Welcome to the club, baby!"*

- Question 11: *"Which membership would you like, Gold or Silver?"*

This is a favorite – the dreaded "A or B" close. Once your rep figures all your objections are out of the way and you're sufficiently enamored with the club, they'll go for the jugular. By giving you limited choices and no perceivable "out," many people cave in. Picture a big, scary cop pulling you over and saying, *"Do you want a speeding ticket or a moving violation?"* You'd be too intimidated to ask, *"Can you just let me off with a warning?"*

In this scenario, I'd recommend you say, *"I'm really not sure. I'd like to think about it and I promise I'll call you tomorrow with my decision. Is that okay with you?"*

I guarantee the rep isn't going to be happy, especially if they think they've got you on the ropes. But at least they'll respect your honesty (or pretend to). And that brings us to that *most* hated of client objections . . .

"I want to think about it."

Salespeople *hate* when clients say that, and many don't know how to respond. The perfect escape clause, right? *Wrong.* Hardened reps won't let you get away so easily. They'll come back at you with, *"That's great, John. It's a big decision, and one you absolutely should give some thought to. Maybe I can help you. What exactly is it that you want to think about?"*

Once you've responded to that question – whether your answer is affordability, level of commitment, the commute, etc. – you're back in the ring for round two.

The easiest way to escape an aggressive sales rep is to tell them from the beginning, *"I'm not signing up today. I'm checking out all the area gyms before I make my decision, and you're the first one on my list. Once I've seen them all I'll make up my mind."*

You'll probably hear, *"Well, at least you started with the best,"* as they deluge you with price closes (*"But if you* don't *join today you'll lose the special . . ."*), and other high-pressure tactics. But, if you stick to your guns, that should help get you out of there alive.

SURVIVAL TIP #10

Keep this in mind: even though their goal is to manipulate you into paying them as much as possible, health club sales reps have nothing personal against you – they don't even know you. So for them it's just business.

That doesn't mean you should take the most expensive package just to get the hell out of there. Pressure is pressure, and we all deal with it. However, now when you go into a gym to discuss joining, at least you'll know what to expect.

Most importantly, don't allow yourself to be intimidated. In the end, your choice to join is up to you. The place certainly isn't going anywhere, and there are always sales to take advantage of. If you're happy with the club and the deal, and if it's in your budget and you're ready, then join. If you're not, then don't.

It's that simple. When all's said and done, it's a free country, and the ultimate decision is yours.

CHAPTER 8:

THE SELLING PROCESS, PART 3: "I AM SPARTACUS"

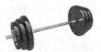

Now that you've learned a little about fitness sales tactics, let's focus on a few examples.

Although the battles fought in sales offices (usually) take place in the mind, when I walked through the doors of my club, I felt like a gladiator entering the gates of the arena. I never knew what my opponents would be like or what tactics I'd have to use against them.

What follows are some unusual closing techniques, riotous instances when my clients managed to turn the tables on me, and a brief glimpse into the cutthroat competition between salespeople.

Remember: in the end, winner takes all. *"There can be only one."*

PULL NO PUNCHES

"Brass," my former manager from Caveat Sports, was the boldest salesman I ever worked with. He pulled no punches and would say anything to anyone. One day, I watched him show a thickset Italian fellow around.

Let's call the guy "Tony."

Tony was very personable and outgoing; he bragged about his new car, his businesses, and the money he was making. Per his doctor, his health was on the line because of his weight – his joining would be a foregone conclusion.

When Brass got him back to the office and told him the total was $1,000.00, Tony's zeal suddenly evaporated. He made up a whole list of excuses about how he had to send his ex child support, buy his kids stuff, give his girlfriend money . . .

Brass was unfazed. He leaned forward in his seat, looked Tony in the eye, and said, "But Tony . . . you're a fat *fuck*. You *gotta* join!"

Tony's face turned contemplative. A second later, he reached for his wallet. "You're right. What do you want, cash or plastic?"

I don't know if I'd ever stick my neck out that far to make a sale. But, it just goes to show, when you establish rapport with someone, *anything's* possible.

CLOSE CALL

Although I was capable of closing clients by playing with their heads, I usually preferred to rely on my sense of humor.

It was a powerful selling tool. Let's face it, you're not going to feel as pressured by someone if you have tears of laughter running down your cheeks (the top set). No one *ever* turned me down once I had them cracking up. I was no longer "Max the sales guy," a potential enemy. I became "Max, their funny pal and soon-to-be drinking buddy."

No wonder I got invited to party with my members all the time.

Inevitably, sometimes it got me into trouble. I had a bad habit of poking fun at myself whenever I did something idiotic by making what I called my "retard noise" (I can hear the politically incorrect uproar now). I'm sure you can imagine it – that uncomfortable, groaning sound that a mentally handicapped person makes when they're frustrated. I even added flailing hand gestures to go with it, God forgive me. Sure, it was horribly insensitive. But at least I was directing it at myself.

One day, two men came in to join. Let's call them "Vito" and "George." They were really cool, down-to-earth guys from the neighborhood, and both had great senses of humor. We were laughing it up in my office, joking about babes and biceps. As we spoke, I discovered that Vito suffered from multiple sclerosis. Mentally he was sharp as a tack, but physically he was impaired. He had a tough time walking, and when he spoke, well . . . forgive me for saying it, but he sounded retarded.

For some reason, in the middle of doing their contracts, I found myself all thumbs. I tried three times in a row to put Vito's phone number in the computer, and each time I screwed up. After the fourth attempt, I got so annoyed I threw up my hands – and *guess* what came out of my mouth?

You got it.

I had a heart attack. I realized my self-deprecating sound effects could only be interpreted one way – as me making fun of poor Vito because of his condition – and in front of his cousin, no less. I was 100% right. Their eyes opened wide in shock and fury. I felt two inches tall; I was *so* embarrassed and ashamed, and the worst part was that I *liked* these guys (in a strictly heterosexual, fellow-gym-dude kind of way, of course).

I was too terrified to look them in the eye; sweat ran down the back of my neck as my heart pounded in my ears. Believe me, if there was a back door to that office, I'd have been through it like a missile. I didn't know *what* to do, so I just kept rambling and typing. I have no recollection what I was babbling about – it could have been the assorted sub-species of crab lice in Beijing, for all I know. After a few minutes of this onslaught of insanity, I finally saw them relax. They undoubtedly realized it was an unintentional slip on the part of the village idiot, and graciously let it slide.

Editor's Note: no joke, I aged ten years from that experience.

HAVE YOU NO SHAME?

Gym salespeople will sign up just about anyone in order to get a commission but I once signed up someone who actually *was* mentally handicapped. In my defense, I had no idea at first.

For purposes of this book, his name was "Elvis."

When I first met him, Elvis seemed a little odd. He was obviously very gay (based on his speech and mannerisms), but it took me a while to catch on that he also had the mind of a ten-year-old. It wasn't until I spotted his Scooby Doo backpack that I realized something was amiss. I was going to back out of the sale, but my manager at Empirical Sports needed numbers and forced me get on the phone and speak with Elvis's mother.

Devil that I was, I convinced her it was a good idea for him to exercise and interact with other people. She hesitated, but eventually went for it.

To be fair, I had no idea what antics I'd be stirring up by throwing a mentally challenged gay man into a locker room full of Bensonhurst muscleheads. Innocent though he was, Elvis had strong sexual urges that he didn't know how to cope with. Soon, he started approaching men in the locker room and saying and doing unusual things.

Normally these "tough guys" would punch a gay guy in the nose for propositioning them, but word quickly spread about the "mentally-challenged-homo" working out there, and I guess people felt guilty getting angry and blowing up at him. Either that or they just didn't know how to respond to his advances.

But boy, did *I* hear about it.

One day, a lynch mob came charging into my office, accusing me of being the "son of a bitch" who signed up the "gay retard." One of them was a 300 lb. bodybuilder. He complained that Elvis had come up to him while he was changing, asked him how he got his chest so big, and wanted to know if he could touch it. Another guy said that Elvis yanked back his shower curtain, asked him if the water was hot, and offered to scrub his back.

The funniest one, though, came a few days later. Two middle-aged male members were chilling out in the Jacuzzi. All of a sudden, Elvis pranced in, naked as a jaybird – sporting an impressive erection. He walked right up to them and yelled out, "Hi guys . . . how's the water? Mind if I join you?" Still "at attention," he stepped boldly into the hot tub. The two men (let's call them "Jake" and "Bentley") screamed in collective horror and, well . . . have you ever seen that nature documentary where the polar bear attacks a bunch of walruses on an ice floe? The bear pounces on the nearest fat, juicy walrus and tears at it, then moves on to another. And all the while, the remainder of the herd flees for their lives, waddling off to either side like the Red Sea parting.

That's exactly what happened in my Jacuzzi. These big, stocky men screamed and fled, clambering clumsily out of the back of the hot tub – where there are no exit steps, I might add – while poor Elvis sat there at periscope depth, smiling confusedly.

It's far from professional, but I laughed about this for days.

Unfortunately, the ongoing entertainment Elvis provided was doomed to end. One day, he took a dump in the men's sauna and smeared excrement all over our wooden benches. Coupled with the extreme heat, you can imagine the smell. Embarrassed, he came out of the sauna and rinsed out his feces-soaked towel in the sink, clearing out the remainder of the locker room in the process.

I had no choice. I was forced to contact his mother and revoke his membership.

What can you do? *Shit* happens.

THE BOWELS OF DESPAIR

Once, I was closing a sale at Empirical Sports. I'd just finished sealing a deal and was putting my new client's membership in the system. He was a cool dude in his early twenties, fired-up to start training. I was just about done when, all of a sudden, a middle-aged woman burst into my office.

"There is *SHIT* all over the women's locker room!" she screamed.

"Excuse me?" I replied.

"You heard me," she shrieked, waving her hands wildly about. "There is shit – *human* shit – all over our locker room!"

Besides being caught off guard by this unexpected assault – the woman (let's call her "Cat") had been a loyal and reserved client for a decade – I dreaded the effect this was going to have on my sale (I was just reaching for the guy's credit card).

Relentless, Cat kept jumping up and down and screaming about fecal matter. And all the while, I stared at her like she was out of her mind (which wasn't far from the truth).

When Cat finally noticed my utter lack of comprehension, she calmed down. "Weren't you here yesterday?" she asked.

"No," I said. "I don't work on weekends."

"Oh. Well, yesterday the sewer pipe in the women's shower area exploded, and they didn't clean it up!" she said, foaming at the mouth. "There is *shit* all over the place. It's on the walls, the shower curtains, the ceiling . . . There's *dried shit* all over the place!"

I stared at her like a deer in headlights. Finally, I managed a feeble "Thank you?" then, before she could start ranting again, hastily added, "I'll, uh . . . mention it to the manager and make sure it gets addressed."

Cat sucked in a deep breath, rolled her eyes, and then stormed out of my office. I was afraid to say anything, dreading what was to come. Finally, I turned to my assuredly-about-to-cancel client and ventured, "Sorry about that, dude. This type of thing doesn't normally go on around here . . ."

To my amazement, the kid grinned and said, "Oh, it's no problem. I don't care. It's not like it's the *men's* locker room!"

What could I say at that point, except thank *God* for male chauvinists.

EXPECT THE UNEXPECTED

Price presentations can go awry. One day, back when I was still a trainer at Caveat Sports, I watched in astonishment as a middle-aged Italian gentleman went berserk and attacked his salesman in the guy's office. The rep had inanely reached over and touched his wife's leg, flirting with her in an effort to convince her to join, too. It didn't go over well. Even though the husband was in his late fifties, it took both the club manager and me to hold him back.

And the woman chose not to sign up.

A colleague once was pricing a particularly harried housewife. In the heat of negotiations, the woman's two-year-old daughter stood up, dropped her drawers, and sank down into a full squat. The look of sheer horror on my peer's face was priceless as she stuttered, "W-what's she doing? She's not going to . . ."

A moment later, the darling little cherub took a shockingly huge dump on my co-worker's floor. And five seconds after that, I was in Hoboken – lest some fool try to ask *me* to clean that shit up. And I mean that *literally*.

I once spent twenty minutes trying to close a client I fondly refer to as *"The Boogie Man."* He had a disturbing habit of picking his nose. And we're not talking regular, old-fashioned digging for gold. This dude had a proboscis like a tapir and had at least two thirds of his index finger up there as he tried to haggle with me. Every so often he'd extract the finger, check it and wipe it on his shirt, then shove it back up his nose and continue excavating.

I didn't know *what* to do. I finally gave him whatever he wanted, just to get him the hell out of my office. To top it off, when we were done, he tried to shake my hand. I stared, horror-stricken, at that outstretched, five-digit shovel of his, like he had leprosy.

"Um . . . that's okay. I'm good."

Come to think of it, that just may be the best way ever to get a good deal on a membership. Just do something utterly disgusting while negotiating. You could shove your hand down your pants and scratch your crotch (sniff your hand once in a while, too), pull out a mirror and pop your zits . . . hell, the sky's the limit. Your frazzled sales rep will forget their entire game plan and throw you the best deal possible, just to get rid of you.

Wow. The Boogie Man was a genius.

DEEP THOUGHTS

A very charming young lady named "Broadway" used an equally astonishing, albeit slightly less ingenious, distraction technique on me at Empirical Sports.

Broadway was an opera singer from the city, and she was a BBBW (Big Black Beautiful Woman), as they call them. For some reason, girls like that always like me. I guess I must look like a life-sized Ken doll and they want to take me home and play dress-up or something.

I was crunching her membership numbers, my fingers tapping nimbly away on my calculator, when I noticed her giving me this peculiar, almost studious, look. Out of nowhere she said to me, "You know, you're kinda cute. If you *want*, I'll get under your desk and suck your dick right now."

I blinked as reality took a vacation. There'd been no flirting, no sexual innuendos flying around. There was *nothing*. I was positive I'd somehow misheard her.

"W-what did you say?" I stammered.

"Oh, you *heard* what I said," she said, smiling hungrily. "But you can't move around a lot, cause we'll get *caught*."

My mind reeled. After a moment, I rested my palms on my desk and pushed my chair back and away, staring down at the woefully inadequate space underneath. "Man, this crazy woman wouldn't even *fit* under my desk!" I thought (not that I was considering it).

I pulled my chair back, hands still on the desk, then leaned forward and gave her a smile. "Thanks," I said. "But, I'm gonna have to pass."

"Suit yourself," she purred.

"Sorry."

"Rain check?"

"I don't think so."

Despite Broadway's attempt to make me think with the wrong head, I stayed focused and got her to join. She wasn't the type to give up easily, though. The next day, she left me tickets for her show at the front desk, along with a note that said she was curious to see if I'd be "impressed with her vocal range."

I have no idea what that meant.

For the record, just because I didn't let Broadway get under my desk, doesn't mean I'm a saint; remember who we're talking about. I'm as capable of succumbing to temptation as the next guy, and probably the guy after that, too. It just depends on whether the risk is worth the reward.

And, of course, I'd prefer not getting *fired* over it.

CORONARY

A similar incident at U. S. Fitness damn near cost me my job and gave me a heart attack. I have to admit that over the course of my career I've done a lot of unsavory things. But *this* one, however unplanned, was absolutely insane.

I'd just signed up "Jessica," a very attractive blonde girl from Brazil. It was an amazingly easy sale. I just recommended a package, and she smiled as she handed over her credit card.

I didn't realize the negotiations weren't over.

Jessica had apparently just come from happy hour. She had on a micro-skirt and I could smell the tequila on her breath from all the way across my desk. No sooner had she signed her contract than she tried getting frisky. She stood up, sauntered around my desk, and started straddling me. At first, I was too stunned to move, not sure what was happening.

The next thing I knew, she pulled her top up and shoved her tongue in my mouth. I was going to go along with it, but the doorknob to my office started to turn. I hadn't expected a "sales bonus" of this kind, so I'd left my door unlocked. My boss, "Britney," had just cracked my door (and gave me an aneurysm), when a member stopped her and asked her a question. That unexpected miracle gave me just enough time to shove a wildly panting Jessica under my desk and out of sight.

Boy, was *that* a mistake.

Based on my personal experience, Brazilian women are far from shy; in fact, they're tigresses. No sooner had my boss sat down across from me, when I felt Jessica undoing my zipper. I guess she must have figured my little buddy down there needed CPR, because before I could mouth the words "Oh God!" she started giving him mouth-to-mouth! I couldn't believe what was happening. I was helpless and trapped. It was incredibly erotic, yet beyond scary. My fear made things so exciting that I got as hard as an Olympic weight bar, but I was also so worried about getting caught that there was no way I could finish.

Which was probably just as well – I don't think I could've handled that.

I sat there, pretending to listen to everything Britney was saying, while Jessica kept going like a rabbit in a battery commercial. Sheets of sweat ran down the back of my neck and soaked through my shirt. Worse, every so often the girl would come up for air, opening her jaws to adjust her python's grip, and make this low, sucking sound. To cover up what was "going down" I pretended I was badly congested, making loud, sniffling sounds and clearing my throat.

All the while, Britney, oblivious to my plight, kept rambling about sales, quotas, and other budgetary nonsense. I can guarantee she never got more emphatic agreements from anyone in her life. Everything she asked was met with a resounding "Sure!" or "Yes!" or "Damn straight!"

When Britney finally got up to leave, she paused in my doorway and glanced back at me. My heart stopped – I thought she'd figured out what was going on. Thankfully, she hadn't. She just pursed her lips, gave me a nod of approval, and left.

I waited a few seconds before freeing myself from Jessica's grip and cursed her out for "putting me in that position."

Then I hobbled over and locked my door.

SURVIVAL TIP #11

This is for both health club members and employees. As wildly arousing and entertaining as that last section was (at least for me), given the choice, I would never have initiated it.

It's not a matter of not being interested; it's about survival – job survival. Over my years in the industry, I've seen dozens of people get caught having sex in gyms, and I know of scores more. I personally caught people I knew "in the act" (and said nothing), and ignored others because I didn't want to expose or interrupt them.

Call it professional courtesy.

With those latter exceptions, however, everyone caught bumping uglies in one of my clubs was fired or thrown out on the spot. So if you value your club or your job, take my advice: there really is a time and place for everything, so keep it in your pants until then. Getting busted is embarrassing and makes you look classless (said the pot to the kettle).

And trust me, it's hard paying for a motel when you put your hand in your pocket and all you feel is your leg.

NO GOOD DEED . . .

Sometimes, trying to be nice comes back to bite you.

When I was doing sales at Empirical Sports, I once signed up a well-known porno star. And when I say porno star, she was the real deal. She'd made *hundreds* of movies, with both men and women. Up close, you could kinda tell. Still, she was eager to join and seemed like a nice person. Plus, of all people, I was hardly in a position to judge. I gave her a good deal.

A few days later, "Shy" bounced into my office and asked me for a favor. She said she needed to catch a bus a half-mile away, and the street outside was long, dark and scary. She said she was afraid to walk there because of the way she was dressed, and asked me to drive her.

The gym was dead at the moment, so I agreed. As I pulled out of the parking lot, I heard her say, "So . . . what do you think?" I turned to find her top pulled up and her big silicone breasts exposed. My eyes peeled wide and I blinked to make sure I wasn't seeing things.

"Uh . . . very nice." was all I managed.

"Wanna touch them?" she asked. Before I could say anything, she grabbed my right hand and slapped it on her left tit. Being a guy, I wasn't about to pull away. So I sat there, driving with my left hand and "turning the radio knob" with my right, all the while praying no cop was waiting to ambush people at the end of the block.

As I turned under a nearby overpass and kept going, Shy gave me a surprised look. She assumed, after handing me one of her boobs, that I'd be turned on and pull over for a quick blow job.

That wasn't happening.

When I got to her bus stop she sat there, waiting for me to make a move. When I didn't, she asked why. I told her I was in a relationship and wasn't interested. Her response was (and this is a direct quote): "Oh, c'mon, Max. You know you want to taste me."

All joking aside, I gagged and very nearly hurled on the spot. *Taste her?* I'd rather gargle with razor blades – it would have been safer.

I politely declined her generous offer, but she wasn't used to rejection. She sat there, stunned. Then she got out, gave me a pissed-off look that translated to: *"You gay mother-fucker . . ."*, slammed the door, and went on her way.

I drove quietly back to my club. When I walked in, I sprinted into the men's room and washed my hand three times, then added a layer of hand sanitizer, just to make sure.

DEALING WITH COMPETITORS

When aggressive salespeople work together, a degree of competition is inevitable. Greedy and unscrupulous reps will take advantage whenever they can, taking any chance to grab an easy commission. In the wake of such thievery, verbal and physical confrontations are common.

To promote peace and harmony in the workplace, I always tried to find alternative ways to exact revenge on my co-workers without resorting to threats, violence, or going to management.

It just took a little creativity.

Once, when I was managing a Caveat Sports in the city, "John," the manager of one of our sister clubs, stole two of my clients. We were on equal footing, and policy-wise, I had no means of obtaining justice. So I decided to invoke a rather unorthodox method of retaliation.

I had a personal trainer working for me named "Cedrick." Cedrick was a short, unassuming-looking guy, but he was the most vocally gifted individual I've ever known. He could do uncanny impersonations of people – movie stars, comedians, politicians – you name it. His favorite routine, however, was calling people and pretending to be a fictitious gay lawyer named "Hiney Lichtenstein."

It's impossible to give "Hiney's" lisping voice any justice via writing, so you'll have to use your imagination. I closed the door to my office, put him on speaker, and had him call my unsuspecting colleague. Their conversation went like this:

Receptionist: "Caveat Sports, how may I help you?"

Hiney: "Hi, can I speak to John, the manager, please?"

Receptionist: "Sure, may I ask who's calling?"

Hiney: "This is Hiney Lichtenstein. I'm a client."

John: "Hi, this is John. Can I help you?"

Hiney: "Hi, John. This is Hiney Lichtenstein. You signed me up a few weeks ago."

(John couldn't remember anyone he enrolled yesterday, so he automatically assumed everything was on the up-and-up).

John: "Sure. I remember. What can I do for you?"

Hiney: "Well, John, I was doing those exercises you told me about the other day. You know, for legs?"

John: "Okay . . ."

Hiney: "Something went wrong and, well . . . I think I hurt my ass."

John: "Your . . . *what*?"

Hiney: "Yeah, I must have pulled something. My ass is on fire! It's one big knot. Maybe there are some stretches we can do together to loosen it up? Or maybe we could meet me in the sauna and you could rub some lotion on it for me?"

John: (horrified) "Excuse me?"

Hiney: "It's terrible. Also, my hemorrhoids are *killing* me. They're all swollen and lumpy and –"

John: "*CLICK!*"

After that, John tried dodging Hiney's phone calls by hiding behind his receptionist, but that only resulted in Hiney getting his dander up. He flamboyantly cursed out the front desk girl, telling her he was a high-powered attorney and that the manager had promised him he'd sit in the steam room with him. *Now*, John was dodging his calls. He had *better* call Hiney back *or else...*

By the time Hiney was done screaming at her the girl was shaking.

It *is* a round world, though.

A co-worker once got even with me after I gave him a work-release prison convict as his walk-in. Personally, I didn't see what the problem was. Sure, the guy was a convicted drug dealer, but it wasn't like I didn't want him to join. I did. In fact, I told my colleague we'd call his package a "workout-release" membership, just to give it a little zing.

My colleague decided to retaliate. The next day, he sent me these two huge transvestites as prospects. And these girls were *scary*. Besides being in full drag, they were both 6'5" (6'10" with heels), 270 lb. competitive body-builders. Shaking hands with them (they gave me delicate, princess-style handshakes) was like grabbing a big bunch of bananas.

Taking them on a tour certainly turned heads. And when we got near the locker rooms, I didn't even stop. There was no *way* I was dealing with *that* issue. I just turned around and brought them back upstairs.

Editor's Note: I guess it's like that old saying goes – some days you're the pigeon and some days you're the statue.

CHEMICAL WARFARE

When waging war with competing sales reps, I used every weapon at my disposal. Let's be frank, gym life is a bit coarser than life on the "outside." Being a typical male on a high protein diet, and having an athlete's high-octane gastro-intestinal system, I sometimes made use of what I'll refer to as *gaseous anomalies*.

One day at Caveat Sports, my colleague "Pack" was lurking by the front desk while I used the restroom. As luck would have it, a well-dressed family of three came prancing in. It was my turn for an up. But since I wasn't physically present, Pack was technically within his rights to snatch them up.

He did, and when I showed up, he smirked in my face.

I can't speak for all club salespeople, but most of the ones I've known (myself included) can be petty when they lose a sale that way – especially one with such a large commission. I knew that Pack's routine would include a tour of the gym floor before he priced them, so I decided to leave him a nice thank-you gift.

I'd had a particularly virulent chili-cheese-dog for lunch that day, and oh, was it barking. I snuck into Pack's office and unleashed an olfactory explosion that would kill most men. Then, to make sure it didn't escape, I shut his door tight and went into my office to practice my innocent expression.

A few minutes later, Pack came strutting by with his clients, his chest puffed out and a smug look on his face. I watched in anticipation as he opened his office door. I heard him say, "Let's all step in here and–"

Pack's eyes popped and he stopped cold. The people behind him piled up like derailing train cars, plowing one into another. He stepped back, slamming his door tightly shut. "Uh, let's use this office instead . . ." he murmured as he herded them back toward the front, discreetly flipping me off behind their backs.

I used a similar technique to get some payback on Dillinger, the first sales rep I worked with, who used to steal my sales by telling clients I'd quit the gym and joined the army. Finally, an opportunity came where I could exact some revenge.

It was a day when downing a whole bottle of Beano wouldn't make a difference. I just kept ripping searing-hot, silent killers. My poor office chair, impregnated with foulness, took on a life of its own. No matter what I sprayed it with, nothing got rid of the stench. Even airing the room out didn't help. The chair was the root of the problem – the moment you plopped down on it: *Poof!*

Our chairs were all identical, so I waited until Dillinger went to lunch and made the switcheroo. A short time later, he took a couple of prospects into his office. I crept by, pretending to check on a nearby wall poster so I could relish the goings-on. Soon, everyone in the room had recoiled in disgust. My mission was a success.

A few minutes later, the couple left and Dillinger came right at me.

"Okay, what the hell did you do to my office? It smells like hell in there!"

"What?" I replied as innocently as possible. "What are you talking about?"

"As soon as I sat down, this God-awful smell filled the whole room. It was like a bomb went off!" He shook his head in disgust. "They were looking at me like *I* did it!"

"Hmm, let's see . . . obviously I wasn't in the room . . . which means it was just you three. Are you sure it wasn't you, or maybe one of *them*?"

"I'm telling you, it was *you!*" he shrieked. "You ruined my sale!"

"I wasn't even *there*! Did they join?"

"Hell, no," Dillinger muttered. "They couldn't wait to leave."

"Sorry, pal." I shook my head as I walked away. "Better luck next time."

I was a real stinker back then.

IN A HANDBASKET

Speaking of things blowing up in your face . . .

One lesson I learned the hard way is that a successful close doesn't always end up as a sale. Sometimes less is more. Once you've got the sale, it's better to leave well enough alone and keep your big mouth shut.

Especially if you're as loquacious as I am.

I was finishing up signing "Dante," a silver-haired Baptist minister, at a Caveat Sports in NYC. The negotiations were over and the sale was closed – just the paperwork was left. I printed up Dante's contract and handed it to him to sign. He scanned the document, and then asked what some of the fine print meant. I felt a sudden twang of uneasiness as I opened my mouth to tell a joke, but I ignored it.

I shouldn't have.

I already knew that Dante was a deeply religious man who took sin and its ramifications very seriously. Yet despite this, I ignored my instincts and told him the same disarming joke I'd used on thousands of people.

"Oh, you know, Dante . . . the usual stuff. Your first-born belongs to us, soul burns in hell for all eternity, yada, yada, yada . . ." To my astonishment, a crazed look came over Dante. He screamed and, before I could stop him, ripped his contract into a dozen pieces. Still yelling, he sprang to his feet and ran out of there like the place was on fire, ignoring my protestations as he went.

Religion and politics – two things you should never discuss, even in a gym.

SHAME ON ME

My most bizarre close was also the most entertaining. I was working at U.S. Amazing Fitness, and was trying to sign up an attractive, albeit demure, young woman. I'd been waiting for a client worthy of trying an experimental new technique on, and this girl was perfect.

As we went over membership prices, I deliberately focused on the most expensive plan we had.

"It's only $949.00 for the year," I said. "Isn't that great?"

Her eyes widened. "Wow . . . it's "$949.00?"

"Yes," I replied. "Do you finger your ass a lot?"

She blinked in surprise, then her eyes bored angrily into mine. "What did you just say?"

With absolute calmness, I replied, "I said, do you figure we *ask* a lot. For the membership? You seem surprised."

Completely confused, she fidgeted in her seat, her eyes moving furtively around my office. "Oh, no . . . it's uh, fine. I'll uh . . . take the basic package."

"Suit yourself."

As I punched in her data, I watched her out of the corner of my eye, all the while praying for the strength to maintain my poker face. I felt sorry for the poor thing. From her body language and rapidly-changing expressions, she must have been thinking, *"Did he really just say that? Did I imagine it? Am I horny? Do I need to get laid? Am I getting my period? Maybe I'm pregnant?!?"*

As she walked out of the club, clutching her contract and trying to remember the name of her therapist, I finally let loose, guffawing until my ribs hurt.

Yes, I'm the devil.

But at that point in my career, I couldn't help it.

Editor's Note: My colleague Pack foolishly tried running my gambit on someone the next day. He blew it. His timing was off, he screwed up his lines, and, when cornered, he completely lost his composure. He literally groveled to keep his victim from getting him fired. Luckily, she liked him and saw the humor in it, so she cut him a break.

Pack told me afterward that it was the scariest thing that ever happened to him.

I considered it to be justice from on high – payback for those two Godzilla-sized trannies the bastard sent me . . .

CHAPTER 9:

CAVEAT EMPTOR

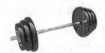

or the uninitiated, *caveat emptor* is Latin for: "*Let the Buyer Beware.*" It's common sense for just about any purchase, but based on what we've learned so far, when it comes to buying a health club membership, even more so.

You've gone through the entire sales presentation. You've done the meet-and-greet, told your rep your reasons for wanting to join, seen the place, gone over pricing, and negotiated a decent package for yourself. You're done. You've survived the worst of it and you're home free, right?

Maybe . . . maybe not . . .

If I was a betting man, I'd wager on *not*.

Just how far will salespeople go to make a commission, and what will they do to keep it? What about your actual contract? Was it thoroughly explained? Do you understand it and have you read the fine print? Do you know what everything means before you sign off on it? Are there any catches or clauses you need to worry about? Are there any questions you haven't asked that you should?

Over the course of this chapter, I'm going to focus on those points, and more. We'll delve into the most important parts of contracts – the parts most sales reps don't want their clients to know. We'll talk about restrictions, hidden charges, follow-ups, dealing with customer service, and making sure you're getting the most for your money – hopefully, with the least amount of grief.

SUPPING WITH THE DEVIL . . .

It never ceases to amaze me what health club sales reps are capable of – and a lot of it is learned behavior. My sales training set the foundation for my future actions. Of course, the instructors only taught us things that were merely unethical.

The illegal stuff we learned on the job.

In my first few months of selling I was exposed to a barrage of shady sales tactics. The turnover rate in my gym (and in every gym I worked) was incredibly high. Most salespeople only lasted a month or two before they got fired, so I had to deal with one character after another.

Why were salespeople terminated so often? Because of the things they said and did. Ethically speaking, I found them to be among the worst, ranking right alongside used-car salesmen. In fact, a few of them actually *were* used-car salesmen, prior to coming to my club. I saw them lying to and cheating clients, and as a trainer, I often cleaned up after their empty promises.

Frankly, they were the reasons I was hesitant about doing sales in the first place.

I have to admit that, in the end, I became as guilty as any of them. It was inevitable, although it did take awhile. When I started doing membership sales at Caveat Sports, they took me aside and taught me the club's under-handed tricks. Each club has its own list of tactics, and the reps at any given location pass that knowledge on to the next generation.

They are breeding grounds of villainy.

For example, we used to offer family-add-on memberships: if a couple joined together, their combined rate was cheaper on a per-person basis. If the primary member paid $50.00 per month, and the spouse paid $20.00, it was $70.00 total, or $35.00 per person. If you added a child or two, it was lower still. It was a great way to rack up numbers, especially for people to whom price was an issue. True, the commissions were lower, but the actual sales numbers looked great on paper.

To keep the staff honest, we had to attach proof of relationship to these contracts, especially if the last name was different. Over the years, the salespeople there had accumulated marriage licenses and birth certificates from all over the world. The valuable originals were photocopied, and then the data (names, dates, signatures), on the copies were covered over. The resultant copy was a blank document waiting to be abused.

Birth certificates weren't the only things they altered. Using the same methods, I watched my colleagues make changes to IDs (DOB, last name) which – when properly photocopied – were absolutely undetectable. I was amazed. I saw them sign up groups of people numbering five or more at a time – one time *twelve*. And all of them were magically related, even those who were underage.

Long story short, if a couple objected to signing up because of the price, or if they wanted their twelve-year-old daughter to attend, too, where there was a will there was a way.

And some correction fluid . . .

NO NEWS AIN'T GOOD NEWS

Many sales reps like to limit the amount of information they give out to clients about their contract. This is done for two reasons: The first is to prevent the client from discovering things in their contract they might not like (hidden dues, terms, etc.); the second is to prevent them from canceling their membership.

Keeping people from canceling has nothing to do with improving their health and fitness, nor with helping the gym remain in business. It's to prevent the sales rep from being decommissioned, an annoying policy that some of the more frugal health clubs out there abide by. When a client's contract gets canceled within a certain period of time (even for billing problems), the rep's commission for the sale is retroactively taken out of their next check.

With the exception of trial-period cancels (wherein the client cancels and gets a full refund), I found decommissions to be deucedly unfair. Typically, the sales rep's cut is more than covered by the member's down payment. Anything after that is profit. So why take away your sales force's hard-earned commissions? They're under enough pressure already without having to worry about getting hit from out of left field. It only makes them more dishonest.

Policies vary, but most clubs decommission for the first three months of any given membership. After that it's free and clear. A notable exception is Caveat Sports. I remember discovering I'd been penalized for sales done *years* prior.

Many gym reps implement an assortment of unethical methods in an effort to cut back on all the bloodletting.

Here are a few of the more popular ones:

Not Explaining Cancelation Policies: A perpetual favorite. State laws require that a gym give its clients a period of time to use their facility to make sure they're satisfied with the purchase (three days is typical). If they're not, they're entitled to cancel for a refund.

If a client doesn't know *how* to cancel, however, the odds they will do so decrease dramatically. Most people, lulled into a false sense of security, don't bother reading their paperwork before signing it. I estimate, of the 25,000-plus people I enrolled, only 10% looked at their contract, and only 1% studied it in detail.

They were lucky that I told it the way it was.

Not Giving a Copy of the Contract: Another classic. By not giving the client the hard copy of their membership agreement, the sales rep stops them from finding out *what* they purchased (including the terms) and prevents them from knowing *how* to cancel. As I said, most clubs require members to cancel within a certain time period by registered or certified mail to their corporate office. Enclosing the member's copy of the contract is often a prerequisite. If the member doesn't have the contract, they have nothing to send and no knowledge of where and how to send it.

Excuses for not giving copies of contracts vary. I read an article in a well-known NYC paper where undercover reporters visited eight different health club chains, including mine. Of the twenty-five places they went to, only my club explained the cancelation policy in full *and* gave a copy of the contract. The other places gave excuses like, "We send all our paperwork to corporate," or "We can't give out a copy because the contracts are all numbered and it would throw off the system."

Editor's Note: for the record, it was me that signed up that undercover reporter. Because of my success rate at that time, I was constantly accused of doing illicit sales, yet in the end, I was the one guy out of eight different chains in five boroughs who was doing his job properly.

Lying About Contracts: a technique used by disreputable sellers since the days of Lucifer. Caveat Sports is probably the most infamous for this since a group of reporters went into their clubs wearing hidden cameras, and put the resultant footage on the news.

I remember cringing as I watched rep after rep lie to prospects. "Oh, you can cancel anytime you want," and "Whenever you want to stop you just call the club and we'll cancel you over the phone. It's easy!" One salesman even had his manager verbally confirm this, just to seal a deal.

The place was doling out three-year contracts you couldn't escape unless you fell in a coma or moved to Guam.

Eventually, Caveat Sports – humiliated after being exposed on national TV – took action. One of their corporate mouthpieces read a statement of how stunned and outraged they were. They claimed that they'd dismissed their dishonest salespeople and managers the moment the evidence came to light.

They were "stunned and outraged?" What about their victims?

JUST SIGN ON THE LINE . . .

There are a few more things you'll want to be aware of before you scribble your John/Jane Hancock. The first ones are "hidden charges" – and there are many to watch for.

- *Down payments/Initiation Fees.* This is an up-front charge the company uses to pay salespeople's commissions and put extra money in their pockets. These fees can often be reduced if one is tenacious. By standing firm and dealing with the manager directly, you can sometimes get away with putting down nothing.
- *Processing Fees.* Known behind closed doors as the "Extortion Fee," this is another name for a down payment. It may seem like a small number (usually $39.00-$49.00), but when you add it to a "discounted" $49.00 initiation fee, you're now putting down a hundred bucks. The most insulting example of this is when a chain runs a "zero to join" promotion that boasts no initiation fee. If you look closely, though, you'll see an asterisk and fine print stating there is still a processing fee. Suddenly, their zero down is really $50 down. So watch out.
- *Hidden Dues.* This is the way many clubs hike up your regular monthly rate. They'll tell you your membership is (for example) $200.00 down and $40.00 per month. But if you study your contract, your monthly fee actually says $48.00 or even $52.00 per month (and that's *before* taxes). When you ask, the difference will be explained as being your "dues" (what you'd pay to renew your membership). Most people buy this without asking: "But if this is what I pay *after* my contract ends, why the hell am I paying it *now*?
- *Auto-Renewing.* A nasty one. Some clubs take advantage of an auto-renew clause built into their contracts. If you fail to give them thirty days notice before your contract ends (again, by certified mail) it automatically renews for another year. Make sure this clause isn't in your contract, or if it is, that you're well aware of it.
- *Bait and Switch.* Many health clubs advertise incredibly low monthly rates to draw in clients (called "the hook"). Once people come in to join, however, they discover that the deal really *is* too good to be

true. Sure, you can join for $9.99 down and $9.99 per month, but you can only come to the gym Tuesday, Thursday and Sunday, between the hours of 10 a.m. and 3 p.m. – pretty much useless unless you're a retiree with an open schedule.

- *Additional Dues.* This is another hook that lures people in with seemingly cheap rates. When people come in to join they discover that, in addition to that low $29.99 per month they're paying, there's a bi-annual dues fee of another $29.99 (billed conveniently to their credit card).
- *Additional Dues X2.* This technique is used by some of the larger chains. Unless you buy their top-of-the-line plan, you'll pay an extra fee every time you visit one of their "sister" clubs. These fees add up quickly.
- *Dues Increases*. Another tactic used by many gyms is to raise your dues every year. Their right to do this is usually spelled out in your contract, in a hard to notice place, and in very fine print. Your dues can go up any time, and there's nothing you can do about it.
- *Editor's Note: it's like my uncle Otis used to say: "You can't always get the elevator, but you can always get the shaft."*
- *Extras.* You'd expect to pay for things like personal training and massages, but a lot of gyms charge a la carte for just about everything else. Aerobics, cycling classes, daycare – even parking can cost you. I remember a client at Empirical Sports whose daughter wouldn't let her out of the house once she walked in the door after work. Since a Caveat Sports was on her way home, she decided to buy a membership there, too, with her plan being to stop there *before* going home. When I asked her about this additional membership, I grew alarmed. Besides $275.00 down and $60.00 a month for 36 months, there was a charge for classes. To her it was nominal – only $5.00 per class. But when I added on her three classes per week, $56.00 per month suddenly jumped to $124.00 – with parking on top of it. A little much for a dirty, crowded place. Luckily, she'd signed up the day she told me about it. I had her cancel immediately. As a single mom with a lot of bills, it made much more sense for her to just drive another two miles.

FEAR OF COMMITMENT

With the exception of paid-in-full (PIF) plans, wherein the purchaser pays the entire term of their contract up front, there are two general types of health club memberships: commit and non-commit. Both are paid on a monthly basis.

When you're choosing a plan, you often have the ability to choose between the two. The commit membership means you're legally obligated for a set period of time (for example, 12 months), after which your membership becomes pay-as-you-go. At this point it can be canceled, usually with pre-set notice (typically 30-60 days). A non-commit membership can be canceled at any time, usually with the same pre-set notice.

Gyms don't like selling non-commit memberships.

Why would they? They want you locked in so they know they're getting their money. Statistically speaking, fewer than 20% of people who join a gym actually end up using it. So why would the owners give you the chance to stop paying if you realize you've made a mistake?

To deter you from buying non-commit plans, most places make their commit memberships more palatable. They have cheaper dues and a lower start-up fee – maybe none. When the sales rep points this out and shows you how much you'll be saving by going commit, you'll be sorely tempted.

Don't be.

Think about this: if 80% of the people that join gyms never go, odds are 4 out of 5 you'll be one of them. But you'll still have to keep paying. So why commit? It may *look* cheaper up front, but let's consider the worst case scenario, the one where you're *not* going to stick with it. I'm not trying to discourage you; I'm trying to be realistic and save you money.

Let's say your commit membership is $49 down and $49 per month, whereas your non-commit is $79 down and $59 per month. On the surface, you'll save $150 for the year. But what if you get busy, injured, or just plain wuss out after a few visits? With the non-commit you can cancel with 30 days notice and end up blowing just $59 to get out of your contract. If you go with the "money-saving" *commit* contract that some slick sales guy talked you into (because he got paid more), you're paying $649 *more* on your year's membership before you can cancel, *plus* another $59 when you do.

Sounds a little pricey to me.

And it is, especially if you're paying for nothing. Once again, I'm not trying to talk you out of exercising. Not taken to extremes, working out is the best thing in the world. But doesn't it make more sense to start with a pay-as-you-go plan, just to make sure you're going to stick with it?

You won't have to feel like someone screwed you without buying you dinner first.

Editor's Note: almost every gym out there allows people with non-commit plans to convert to a commit contract. Why wouldn't they? Once you know working out has become a stable facet of your life, switching might be a good option. Just make sure they don't charge you a conversion fee.

I've become the proponent of a very sad theory about commit contracts – one I believe shows just how effective fitness chains are at manipulating their clients' pride and self-esteem.

Let me tell you how it works.

Caveat Sports makes money by locking people into long-term contracts. Most of their memberships are multi-year plans that convert to renewal dues at reduced rates. You might join for $150 down and pay $60 a month for three years, after which your dues reduce to a "lifetime" rate of only $100 per year.

Most people who use Caveat Sports memberships for the full term of their contract do so because they're either incredibly dedicated, tremendously tenacious (they know they're stuck and want their money's worth), or just don't know any better. And most of those who stay *after* their contract runs out usually can't afford anything else (seniors on a fixed income make up a good chunk of their renewals).

But let's say you're in that 80% that joined and didn't use the gym (Personally, I believe the percentage is significantly higher).

Let's also say that you couldn't get out of your contract, even though you hated the place, and for fear of having your credit ruined, paid for the full three years. Now, you've gotten a notice in the mail that it's time to renew. At this point, many people run for the hills. But a good chunk *will* renew, even though they only went once or twice or maybe even never.

Why?

It's a psychological thing. After shelling out thousands of dollars for nothing, most people realize they pissed away their money. Some openly admit it, whereas others do so only at the subconscious level. Now, these same people are looking at a renewal notice.

And they jump at it.

For three years, they paid $60 a month to *not* go, so paying $100 per annum for the same thing now seems like a bargain. They also don't want to publicly acknowledge that they were hoodwinked, so they present their decision as a smart investment on their part. I've heard things like, "It's there if I need it," or "I hate the place, but for the price I can't go wrong." And this was from people I signed up at Empirical Sports after their Caveat Sports contract was over.

Don't let yourself get roped in and conditioned like that. If you don't sign a three-year lock-in to a place you've never even toured, you'll never have to make that big investment. Why throw away two or three grand, especially in *today's* economy? Why get suckered in at all?

Take my advice, these days even Caveat Sports offers non-commit plans. Think of joining the gym like getting married – only a fool jumps in right away. Start out dating first with *no* commitment. When you feel the time is right, *then* commit. That's when you should take the plunge. And *only* then should you sign on the dotted line.

A three-year contract to a place you hate is like a bad marriage. Except in this case, only one person is getting screwed.

And that's you.

YOU WANT TO HOLD MY <u>WHAT</u>?

So, you've made up your mind which type of membership you want. You checked your contract thoroughly for any hidden nastiness, and formally joined the gym. Well done.

Starting out at a new place can be a little intimidating. There's scores of new machines and hundreds of unfamiliar people. A lot of people, whether excited to share their new club with their comrades, or simply wanting the company of familiar faces, will bring their friends with them as guests.

Immediately upon arriving at the club's front desk, your guests are asked to hand over a piece of photo identification and leave it at the desk, along with a completed guest registration. A lot of people are uncomfortable doing this.

And with good reason.

Holding IDs from guests is a much maligned trick incorporated at health clubs worldwide. After filling out their tour card (and giving their sales rep everything they need to follow up with them via phone, mail and email) they're required to leave a valid local photo ID. If you ask why, officially, holding onto your guests' ID proves they are who they say they are, thus ensuring the safety of club employees, members, and property. People looking to rob lockers won't leave an ID behind, especially their own. Also, if something happens to a guest while they're there (God forbid), the employees will be able to identify them.

But the real reason – and a fairly obvious one – that a guest is asked to leave their ID is that the sales staff can hold it hostage. And despite what you may be told, it *won't* be waiting for them at the front desk. It will be secreted inside the office of a sales rep. And when the guest wants it back, they'll have no choice but to go to said office, where they'll be cordially invited to sit down.

That's when the fun starts.

Sales reps will spend an hour or more trying to bludgeon guests into joining, even if that person has absolutely no interest. It doesn't matter if they said, *"I live in Montana and I'm only here for three days for my mom's funeral,"* the sales rep still won't let up. It's like they have no soul.

I was fairly aggressive when it came to selling. But I learned early on to pick and choose my battles. It made no sense to me to waste time and energy trying to batter someone into submission who was unable to join. All that does is wear me out and make myself new enemies. Frankly, I have enough of those already.

When trying to close resistant or disinterested parties, some salespeople take things to extremes. If they can't finish the job themselves, they subject prospects to the dreaded "T.O.": the *Take Over*. That's when the rep turns you over to a more seasoned and aggressive individual – typically the manager. This is (hopefully) done subtly. "Okay, I understand you're not ready yet. Let me just get you a class schedule to take with you." Suddenly, the sales office door opens and someone else walks in. "Oh, by the way, this is my manager. I wanted to introduce him to you, in case I'm not here when you come back."

If you hear a distinctive ringing in your ears at this point, don't worry. It's not tinnitus, just the start of Round 2 . . .

Personally, I've always abhorred T.O.s. I never relied on them, even in the early days. It ruins any potential bond between rep and client and turns things into a high-pressure, boiler-room type sale. This doesn't mean I've never done them. I *have* taken over sales for other, less experienced reps, and I *have* held many an ID prisoner. However, I always tried to turn it into a harmless joke by taking the ID and telling them, *"I'll be holding this hostage . . . I mean keeping an eye on this for you while you're working out. Come see me after you're done."*

If you have to do something awkward to someone, it's always good to turn a negative into a positive, or at least mitigate things.

And a well-timed wink often goes a long way.

THE FOLLOW-UP

Seven to thirty days after enrolling, you'll usually get a friendly call from the person who signed you up. On the surface, this will be a "courtesy call," with your sales rep checking to see how your workouts are going.

In reality, they're calling to see if you have any more customers for them. Don't be deceived by their friendly demeanor or if they know your name; they probably don't even remember you. They're just calling off a printed sales report that shows everyone they signed up the previous month. If you don't believe me, test it out for yourself. Invent some mythical conversation you had with your sales rep while you guys were bonding. Maybe mention that "race" you're training for, or the weight loss contest you're in. Ask them if they remembered to bring in that article they promised you.

Their answers/excuses should be quite entertaining.

Anyway, back to the follow-up.

When trying to milk members, some salespeople are direct. They'll tell you there's a big special and ask if you know anyone that might want to take advantage of it. If there really is a special, find out what it is; if it's cheaper than what you got, you may be able to convert or cancel and rejoin. If you can't, it gives you something to hold over your rep's head.

Some sales reps use pressure tactics. They'll tell you your free guest passes are about to expire, so you'd better hurry up and bring your friends in. They may even ask you for their names and numbers – and volunteer to call them for you, "so you won't have to be bothered."

The most competent salespeople won't ask for referrals; they'll simply encourage you and ask if you need anything. This is by far the smartest way to go. When people see that you care about them (or at least pretend to) they're *happy* to refer people to you. Pushy, grasping sales tactics like asking clients to feed you their friends and family members are transparent insults to any educated consumer.

It's simple. If you want people to recommend your club, all you have to do is take care of them. If they're happy and getting results, the referrals are inevitable.

CUSTOMER DISSERVICE

Say a problem suddenly crops up at your local health club. It could be anything: a billing issue, an incident on the gym floor, your locker being broken into . . . What if the manager isn't available, or is unable or unwilling to help you? What do you do?

Most people call their club's 800 number. This is especially true with the larger chains that have customer service agents to answer the phones. Smaller, mom-and-pop style facilities usually deal with their clients one on one, and tend to be more customer-oriented and friendly. They have to be; they need your business. The big chains, on the other hand, function more like grist mills; they sign people up and send them on their way.

Despite being a member of a company that services tens or even hundreds of thousands of people, if you have a problem with something, you'll suddenly be very lonely. When I worked at both Caveat Sports and Empirical Sports, calling their 800 number meant being on hold for ten minutes or more, and suffering through the most dreary elevator music and pre-recorded messages imaginable. Half the time, my calls were "dropped," and the rest of the time, the agents I dealt with were both guarded and uncooperative.

And I was an *employee*.

A customer service rep told me that this is done deliberately as a delaying tactic – to discourage people from staying on long enough to voice their problems.

Most of the managers I worked for were also quite adept at shying away from members' complaints, especially if they were billing or cancelation-related. On the other hand, if someone brought in a friend to join, it was quite the opposite. Then, the club manager got so close that he felt like a Siamese twin.

But if you need to vent about a bad experience, don't be surprised to find that same manager MIA. All club managers have their calls screened by their front desk. A quick intercom is all it takes to give you the brush off. The manager might be "in a meeting," "touring the club," "stepped out," or "just left for the bank," to name a few.

The possibilities are endless.

My favorite artful dodger of a manager was Antonia, my former boss at Empirical Sports. She worked early some days and late others. When a member called that she didn't want to deal with, she had her receptionist tell them she'd just left (feeling ill, personal emergency, sick dog, dentist's appointment . . .) and wouldn't be back until the following day. When the caller – understandably impatient at this point – asked for her schedule, the front desk gave them the opposite of what her next shift really was.

Of course, when that same member called back the next day and discovered she'd just left . . .

SURVIVAL TIP #12

When it comes to fitness facilities, what you see is what you get. So look long and hard before you commit, and tour the place inside and out. Check it out during the times you plan on going, especially if you plan to train at rush hour. Pay attention to the clientele. Besides sheer numbers, are they people you'd feel comfortable being around scantily clad, or is the place filled with juice-heads (steroid users) and gorillas? Is it an obvious meat market? Does the locker room seem secure, and is it clean?

Again, most importantly, study your contract before you sign. Have you heard all of the membership options the place has to offer, or just the one that puts the most money in your sales rep's pocket? Check out the fine print and any hidden charges, as well as cancelation and renewal policies.

Last, but not least, be wary of giving out personal information until you're committed to joining. As a salesman, I was always annoyed when clients gave me fake addresses and phone numbers, but in retrospect it was a great survival tool for prospects.

Don't be afraid to slip a pushy health club sales rep your friend's old cell phone number. The same thing applies when it comes to handing them your driver's license. If they claim they need your ID for security, bring it, but bring a photocopy as well and leave that with them. I've done it at car dealerships many times. Tell your salesman you had a bad experience with a competitor who lost your driver's license, and you'd rather not give it up. If he won't let up and you feel uncomfortable, then leave. At least you won't need to get your ID back at gunpoint or, worse, lose it.

Think smart. If the place is run-down, shady, or filled with sketchy characters, why give them your info? Be an educated consumer and be prepared.

Lastly, if you are a member and you're dealing with your company's service or billing department, be patient and always keep your composure – especially if it's regarding money. Health club phone agents work a thankless job and deal with lots of abuse from irate members. As a result, they're easily put off.

Kill them with kindness; they'll be pleasantly surprised, and maybe even helpful.

Consider using email. It doesn't involve sitting on the phone for twenty minutes, and it's a digital paper trail, so you can prove it if they ignore you. If you do call and you're promised something, try to get an email address and a follow-up confirmation.

That way, you have proof. Otherwise, that conversation never took place.

Remember: Caveat Emptor; it's what's for dinner!

CHAPTER 10:
CLIMBING THE LADDER

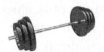

After surviving long enough to prove myself in sales, learning the ins and outs, I began working my way up the slippery rungs of the health club corporate ladder. To put it mildly, I discovered things about my facility I wished I hadn't. I also found out that, when it came to abusing power, I was just as susceptible as anyone I'd worked for. This included my managers, none of whom were examples worth emulating.

For some insane reason, I assumed that things would get better for me as I moved up. That I'd deal with better people, that the job would become less stressful, and that I'd have more over control of my life.

I was wrong. My management peers proved to be just as treacherous, if not more so, than the sales reps. Quotas were higher, and I ended up working even more hours – including on weekends. The view from the top was just as bad as the view from the bottom – maybe even worse.

Editor's Note: In olfactory terms, "you can climb a manure pile as high as you want; the stink always stays the same."

IN NEED OF ASSISTANCE

After the unexpected termination of my predecessor (for many unnamable offenses), I was promoted to Assistant Manager at Caveat Sports. My meteoric rise had less to do with my managerial skills and selling ability than the company's sudden need to fill the position. Regardless, I was not about to complain. With my promotion came money, plus something much more intriguing – something I'd never had before.

Authority.

During the week, the club manager was the big boss, with me working as his immediate subordinate. But I was in charge when he left the club or called in sick (which happened surprisingly often), as well as on Saturdays and Sundays. During the weekends I called the shots, and like most people given a little power, it went straight to my head.

I was no megalomaniacal dictator. My "abuse of power" manifested it-self in more subtle and self-serving ways – linked to whatever I desired at the moment.

Most health club members are frighteningly ignorant of what goes on in their gyms after closing. Abuse of facilities is common; in fact, it's pandemic. As the Assistant Manager I had the keys and alarm codes. I could do whatever I wanted, so why wouldn't I? With the pressure my new position draped across my shoulders, I was working like a slave. I deserved to pamper myself.

So I did.

I initially used my late night isolation for unorthodox purposes. I was a burgeoning fisherman, and would go down to the pool area to practice my casts and retrieves. It was very useful; I could see the action of my lures and readily adjust my technique.

After a few weeks of this, however, I got bored, and started using an entirely different rod . . .

Despite the fact that I had an apartment close by and could take girls home whenever the opportunity "arose," I decided, as Master of my Domain, that I would treat the club like my private estate. I knew my former manager had utilized both the Jacuzzi and men's sauna as his boudoir on numerous occasions – I'd found his condoms and heard him brag about it. And the current manager was doing the same. The only difference was that the new guy was gay, so the condoms I'd find often had additional "evidence" (for want of a better term) on them.

If they could get away with this, surely I could.

Again, we're not talking about during business hours. That would be the shortest route to the unemployment office. This was after closing, when most gym hijinks go on. Sure, during club hours there's plenty of behind-the-scenes activity (robberies, drug use, sex in closets, etc). But it's *after* hours, when nobody can see, hear, or report anything, that staff members in positions of authority take full advantage of the place and milk that cow until its udders hurt.

DOUBLE INDEMNITY

As a former PT, I had a group of devoted female clients who steadfastly refused to give me up. We weren't allowed to combine jobs back then, so I was forced to train them off the books and at odd hours, to avoid getting caught. Regardless of precautions, however, there was always some risk involved. But with the place closed and no one else around, it was an entirely different ballgame.

I had two great gals I loved working with: a demure Jewish girl and a voluptuous Polish girl. Let's call them "Saturday" and "Sunday," because those were the days I saw them. They each came right before quitting time. I'd clear the club, making sure every living soul was out, then lock the place up tighter than Fort Knox. With my paperwork already done and ready to be faxed to corporate, it was up to the gym floor and down to business.

I put each of these girls through an amazing workout (which was easy to do with nobody in the way), for which they paid me cash. Then, with them already pumped, I took them down to the women's sauna for some "post-workout coital conditioning."

Editor's Note: since I knew how at least one of my bosses would abuse the men's sauna, I avoided that place like the plague. The woman's seemed a much safer bet.

Out of pure spite, or maybe to show my disdain for my employers, I'd strip off my condom and hose down the sauna's wooden seats like some x-rated machine gun. Unlike my bosses, however, I didn't want to chance leaving any DNA behind. I smeared my rapidly desiccating goo deep into the wood with my foot, leaving behind a nice, shiny patina that dried rapidly in the intense heat.

There were two great things about my clients riding me in the sauna. The first was they were paying me for PT, so in a perverse way it felt like they were also shelling out for sex, which was a major turn-on. The second was that, after walking out of a hot sauna drenched in sweat, the difference in air temperature was a massive system shock.

For sure, even that couldn't compare to the adrenaline rush of getting caught in the act by the entire population of a local retirement home . . .

CAN YOU SAY . . . U-TUBE?

All things truly do come to an end, and my after-hours adventures at Caveat Sports were no exception. Like my predecessors, I had quite a run, although my playmates certainly weren't limited to paying clients.

The last one nearly cost me everything.

I was dating "Wilomena," a half European, half Asian gymnast who could do a full split between chairs. We really enjoyed one another's company, but one night, our mutual attraction got us into some serious trouble.

We were bored doing it in the sauna, couldn't see in the steam room, and were afraid of catching foot fungus in the showers. So, we went up to the gym floor. After some deliberation, we settled on defiling our club's inner-thigh machine. After all, with Wilomena's insane flexibility, it made sense to take advantage of it.

So there I was, saluting, with a smiling Wilomena lounging back in my inner-thigh machine, her toned legs spread like a waiting banquet. Believe me – that was all the invitation anyone would need. It was awesome, or rather it *should* have been.

Unfortunately, I didn't take into account the trains passing by the windows of the second floor. Normally, this wasn't a cause for concern; the trains usually moved fast and it was fairly dark with the club's lights off.

On this particular night, though, for some mysterious reason the train conductor came to a stop with his cars perched directly outside. I don't know if he saw what was going on and decided to rain on my parade (*the bastard*), or if it was just pure, dumb misfortune.

As I turned my head to the side, I realized I was treating a dozen people to the sight of my muscular white ass. I uttered a high-pitched yelp of fear and then freaked. There was a mad scramble as we threw our clothes on and got the hell out of Dodge. It would have been mighty hard to explain to my employers.

Of course, I had far greater concerns. At least one of the old ladies glee-fully watching had her cell phone in hand, and could have easily found a way to screw both Wilomena and me at the same time.

Not exactly the threesome I've always dreamed of . . .

SURVIVAL TIP #13

Take it on faith – I'm far from the only person to use their fitness facility for extracurricular activities. Lots of unusual things go on in club steam rooms and saunas, both during and after hours. So, if you're going to use them, take some precautions. Whether you wear swimming trunks or wrap yourself in a towel, you'll want a protective layer between you and the wood or ceramic underneath. God-only-knows how often they clean those places. Lounging in dried sweat is bad enough, but do you really want to plop your butt down on who-knows-what-else?

CHARACTER SPOTLIGHT: THE JULLIARD WOMAN

As my club's assistant manager, I quickly discovered that discretion was, indeed, often the better part of valor.

When I wasn't risking my job with my extracurricular activities, I was dealing with customer service issues and would-be members. One of my fondest was someone I'll forever refer to as "The Julliard Woman."

I was relaxing at my desk when my receptionist intercommed me to say that a woman was waiting to sign up. I came bouncing out of my office to greet my prospect – an enthusiastic woman in her late sixties. She said she was a graduate of the famous Julliard School in NYC, and that she was once a ballerina. I went over prices with her and she decided to join.

I started doing Julliard's paperwork, but when I asked for payment, she reached into her pocket and handed me (of all things) a welfare check. I stared confusedly at it, then asked if she had another method of payment. She didn't. I apologized and explained that a welfare check wasn't going to work (I've also declined offers of food stamps, but those are stories for another time). If she couldn't come up with an alternative she couldn't join.

Julliard grew angry. She started ranting and raving that I was biased. Then she took up position in my lobby and started screaming at clients as they strolled in, telling every one of them that the place "sucked" and that they "shouldn't join."

Seeing the maniacal look in her eye, I decided it was time for a strategic withdrawal. I went back in my office, locked the door, and called the police. I saw her running back and forth in the corridor outside my office, alternately screaming, "This place sucks! It sucks, don't join!" and "The Julliard School, the Julliard School!"

My poor receptionist, left alone with this nutjob, begged me to let her in my office, or at least not leave her out there by herself. I laughed uproariously, ignoring her pleas and her assertion that I was an abject coward (like *that* was going to make me leave the safety of my carpet-lined cocoon). As I waited for the cops, all I could hear was cursing and "The Julliard School!" echoing through my office walls.

Two police officers arrived shortly thereafter. The female officer was very nice to my would-be client, and explained that all she had to do was come back with an acceptable method of payment. At that point, I'd be happy to sign her up.

Editor's Note: That was 100% true. I really wanted her money. I couldn't care less about her mental state. What was one more lunatic in an already jam-packed asylum?

I don't know why, but the Julliard woman started arguing with the cops. She refused to leave and insisted on joining. I could tell they were starting to lose patience with her. Finally, the female officer told her pointedly, "Look sweetie, you're disrupting their business and the manager is asking you to leave. If you don't go, we're going to have to lock you up."

Julliard got a malicious look in her eye and asked the woman, "Are you a cop?" When the answer was affirmative, her next words were, "Well then, you know what happens *next*!"

Before I could say *"holy shit!"* this fragile, five foot tall, ninety-pound senior pounced on the lady cop. A frantic struggle ensued, and the officer's male counterpart was forced to join in. Together, they subdued and cuffed Julliard. The last thing I heard as they dragged her kicking and snarling out the door was her shrieking: "The Julliard School, the Julliard School!"

The next day, one of the woman's relatives came by the club to apologize for the incident. Apparently, Julliard was an escaped mental patient who'd stopped taking her meds and wandered off. Naturally, she'd ended up where all the other area psychopaths did.

In my lap.

FEARSOME FACILITIES

As I moved into management I found out things about my facility I was completely unaware of – things I wish I hadn't found out at all.

Sometimes it's better being ignorant.

It's a well-known fact that the most widely used and sought after amenities in health clubs are swimming pools, hot tubs, steam rooms, and saunas. People use them for a variety of reasons – exercising, relaxing and soothing aching muscles, and getting a good sweat that relieves tension and releases harmful toxins through the skin.

As you've already discovered, like many other areas of a club, these amenities are often used for different purposes than they were originally intended.

What I *haven't* told you yet is how ill-maintained they often are. If I'd known that earlier in my career, I'd never have set foot in any of them, let alone gotten naked in them . . .

WATER, WATER EVERYWHERE . . .

Of all the places I worked, Caveat Sports was consistently the most unsanitary. Their swimming pools were the worst: uniformly dark, uninviting-looking bodies of water with either mysteriously foul odors or the acrid smell of excessive chlorine.

Editor's Note: if the water you're about to step in is dark gray in color, stop and think. There's something wrong.

As an A.M., I found out why their pools were so gross. It was near closing time and I was making my rounds, ensuring that everyone had vacated the premises. As I made my way down to the pool area, the lifeguard was performing some sort of service on the pool and hot tub. Pipes sticking from the ceiling dumped water into the pool.

I asked what was going on, and she replied, "I'm just changing the water."

I nodded. "Cool. How often do we do that?"

"Every six months."

". . . Six months!" I gasped.

She chuckled. "I know what you're thinking, but relax. We shock it regularly with chlorine, so it kills all the bacteria."

Still shaken, I made my way topside. Despite her assurances, I remained concerned. Forget all the skin cells and hair follicles floating about – with scores of male and female clients collectively releasing God-knows-what into the pool, there was no *way* that water could be clean. I personally witnessed an elderly member lose control and release a large "floater" into the pool. The other occupants retreated like wildebeests fleeing a hungry croc.

After this happened (and unlike in *Caddyshack*), the powers that be did *not* have the pool emptied, scrubbed down and sanitized. When I made the request I was laughed at. Instead, the offending bowel movement was merely scooped up in a straining net and everyone went back to their business as if everything was completely normal.

BLACK WATER, WHITE DEATH

The pinnacle of Caveat Sports' pool grossness came to my attention at Empirical Sports, when one of my clients (who maintained memberships at both facilities) came into my office. He was pale and shaken, with the look of someone who's narrowly escaped death and lived to tell the tale.

"Hooper" had been swimming in a Caveat Sports pool – something he did often. Being a superb athlete, and with this particular pool measuring only fifteen meters long, he swam many of his laps underwater.

Anticipating where his story was going, I interrupted him. "Let me guess. You couldn't see the bottom?"

"No, I *wish* I couldn't see the bottom."

"I don't get it."

Hooper took a deep breath, let it out slow. "I was swimming underwater, when I saw something on the bottom of the pool."

"Okay . . . what was it?"

"A tampon."

I choked. "What? Are you serious?"

"Yes!" he exclaimed, shaking his head and laughing nervously. "It actually came up off the bottom as I got near it. At first, I thought it was a mouse coming at me. When I realized what it was, I beat it out of there so fast people thought the water was on fire. I'm not kidding. Only a great white shark could have made me haul ass faster for dry land."

"Good God . . ."

Hooper shook his head. "Yeah, I mean, seriously – how big does your pussy have to be for that to just fall out?"

"Never mind *that*," I said with big eyes. "Dude, your *mouth* was in that water!"

He later told me that, although he reported "great white" to the club manager, nothing was done about it for days. The tampon was eventually retrieved, but was never returned to its rightful owner.

As you may imagine, Hooper refused to put even his big toe into their pool from that day forward.

THE BLACK LAGOON

The pool at Caveat Sports was bad, but the hot tub was worse. It was simple physics – more bodies, occupying a substantially smaller body of water, that's also only emptied every six months.

Most of the clients who go into Jacuzzis tend to be older people – seniors. That's because they suffer from arthritis and have more day-to-day aches and pains.

They also have less control of their bodily functions.

Picture a crowd of hairy, old curmudgeons, sitting around commiserating, while pissing and farting into your favorite hot tub, relentlessly adding their own juices to the mix. As I mentioned, gym hot tubs are often abused behind the scenes, and not everyone uses protection. So, you can only imagine what *else* is left behind.

I never bought that "chlorine kills everything" argument my lifeguard threw at me. If that was true, nothing could survive in that water. Yet, it did. At times, the Jacuzzi in Caveat Sports had algae growing above the waterline, and all around its edges. You know the stuff I'm talking about: that greenish slime that grows on the walls of poorly maintained fish tanks. But *this* gunk was growing on a hot tub used by people.

One day, an infuriated Russian client bellowed to me at the top of his lungs that the Jacuzzi was only fit for animals, not people.

After leaving Caveat Sports, I found a web site set up by people who hated the chain.

Editor's Note: you know it's bad when you've got a full-blown web site dedicated to your destruction.

On this site was a posting from a doctor, who explained that, because Caveat Sports changed the water in their pools and hot tubs so infrequently, there was an inevitable build-up of uric acid and ammonia from all the urine discharged. This accumulates over time, visible on the water's surface as nasty-looking foam. The ammonia buildup burns the eyes, bleaches the color out of bathing suits, and makes the skin itch until it feels like it's going to peel off.

Let's be realistic. Shocking a pool or hot tub with chlorine may kill off some of the bacteria, but it won't scrape away layers of algae, nor will it remove the ammonia from all the urine. Ammonia is a liquid; it's going to sit there. So what that means is, after six months of your fellow members relieving themselves in the whirlpool, half of what you're sitting in is their piss.

CHAPTER 11:
LOCKERS – RUNNING THE GAUNTLET

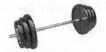

When it comes to confronting unpleasant things in life, many people play the role of an "ostrich." By pretending something doesn't exist, they spare themselves the burden of dwelling on it.

When I was writing *Memoirs of a Gym Rat,* people advised me to do just that, especially when it came to a truly gross aspect of health clubs – locker rooms. As you've undoubtedly realized, though, I'm not shy when it comes to taking on issues.

And this is no exception.

To be fair, many gyms and health clubs have attractive and sanitary locker facilities you might feel very comfortable, even proud using. But an equal number do not. They shirk on cleaning and maintenance, allowing slovenly members to run amok. As a result, their changing areas are, at a minimum, unsanitary, and many have so many blatant health code violations you wonder how they stay in business.

I've seen things in locker rooms that most people can't stomach. I know I couldn't. For your benefit, I'm presenting an abridged version of these experiences.

Even so, if you're like me, and seeing someone clean up after their dog makes you a little queasy, you might just want to do yourself a favor and skip this chapter. If you do that's fine. But remember: just because you don't talk about something doesn't make it any less real.

Especially for the people that have to deal with it.

ROBBERIES (I FEEL <u>VIOLATED</u>)

When it comes to locker rooms, the most important issue is security. Like it or not, most places where people congregate are havens for thieves, and gyms are one of their preferred hunting grounds. It makes perfect sense. Most people who can afford a gym, especially the expensive ones, have lots of cash, credit cards, and jewelry. There's also their fancy cell phone and MP3 player . . .

Locker robberies happened at every place I worked – and regularly. Dinar Fitness hardly had any, but that was most likely because, if you got caught stealing there, the owners might break your legs instead of handing you over to the cops. And smile doing it. Other than that, though, my clubs were like Dodge City.

The first locker robbery I dealt with took place shortly after I became A.M. at Caveat Sports. It was on a weekend, so I had to address it personally. A very upset client of mine came up from the locker room wearing nothing but a towel. Dripping water all over my office, he complained that someone had broken into his locker. They'd taken his wallet (including his entire week's pay), his watch, and even his pants.

I examined the locker in question. Apparently, the victim had used a very small padlock, and all the thief had to do was jam a screwdriver into it and bear down until the clasp broke.

I felt terrible for my client. He was a hard-working guy with two kids and rent that was due. I managed to find him a pair of workout pants to wear on his way home and gave him a few bucks for the train. I also called the police so he could file a theft report and told him I'd call our corporate offices and see what could be done to compensate him.

When I spoke to my boss that afternoon, he screamed at me for calling the cops. I was informed that the company hated documenting thefts (unofficially, of course), and my suggestion to contact the police was not how things were done. Sure, it was fine if the *client* wanted to do it. But I was not supposed to recommend it.

When Monday came around, I called our customer service line. I explained to them what happened and suggested we improve locker room security and compensate the client for his lost earnings and property. The rep laughed at me. He said security cameras in locker rooms were impossible due to legal and privacy reasons. Posting a guard was out of the question – there was no budget for such a thing, let alone any precedent. When I pushed for them to at least compensate the guy, I was told the company wasn't responsible for personal property on the premises, and that there were notices posted to that effect.

I was surprised and annoyed by my company's cavalier attitude and went down to the locker room to see things for myself. I saw no such sign posted, and called back and reported this.

Within twenty-four hours, not only were signs posted in each locker room, stating that the company wasn't liable in the event of a loss, there were large stickers put *inside* each locker saying the same thing.

IT TAKES A THIEF

Locker robberies tend to be cyclical. As in the last example, most break-ins coincide with paydays – especially on Fridays, and the 1st and 15th of each month.

Caveat Sports is notorious for this, and the thieves who roam their clubs are both experienced and organized. One woman used to come in with a key ring loaded with master keys for just about every padlock on the planet. She signed in using a stolen membership card, always right as an aerobics class was about to start. As soon as the locker room was quiet, she'd rob six or ten lockers. And, because she wasn't doing any damage to the lockers or locks, no one knew that they'd been robbed until they cleaned out their locker. Lynch mobs gathered outside my office because I was unable to stop her one-woman crime spree.

Eventually, I caught on to "Caveat's Most Wanted" and her little shtick. The next time "Keys" showed up, I called the police the moment she entered the locker room. The cops took too long, so I followed her as she was leaving. Thankfully, the cops pulled up just as she exited the building. I pointed Keys out to them and they ran her down. Her cries of foul play were quickly silenced when they opened her backpack and found her key ring – plus five women's credit cards and gobs of stolen cash and jewelry.

Funny, Keys never came back after that.

I guess someone finally showed her a lock she couldn't open . . .

As you can see, standard issue padlocks are pretty much useless. Combination locks are a little better, but they aren't a perfect defense either. If you use one, look around to see who's watching, and make *damn* sure you spin the dial after you close it. If you don't, a clever crook can just jiggle it up and down.

In some gyms the type of lock you choose can be meaningless. I've had thieves use miniature bolt cutters or small pinch bars to physically break locks. And if a lock turned out to be too tough, they'd attack the door's hinges. Due to the amount of noise involved, these types usually work in pairs; one acts as a lookout while the other does the deed.

The slickest thieves won't touch your cash. It'd be too obvious, and their crime would be reported. Instead, they'll slip out one or more of your credit cards, and by the time you've finished your workout and gone home, they've already banged you out for five or ten grand. Some of them even put used credit cards of the same type back in your wallet so nothing looks amiss – until you go out to a restaurant and hand the waiter some poor slob's stolen Amex.

Few things in life are more humiliating than being handcuffed and dragged away from your dinner date by the boys in blue.

PREVENTITIVE MAINTENANCE

As I mentioned, if you do get robbed, don't expect any help from management. Naturally, they'll pretend to sympathize with you. They have to. But the truth is they deal with issues like this all the time. Their real goal is to keep you from making a scene (imperiling potential sales). They also want to reduce the chance that you'll report your loss.

At Empirical Sports, locker break-ins reached epidemic proportions. The managers always tried to cover it up. They'd give out clothing from the pro shop to appease violated members and keep them from filing complaints.

Your best defense to avoid being a victim is to take precautions – a lot of them. Start with the obvious: don't bring your valuables to the gym. Sure, that shiny Rolex works wonders on the girls outside, but do you really want to risk scratching it up on a weight bar?

If you do bring valuables, many places have small lock boxes by the front desk. They're hard to open and usually in full view of the reception area, so they're a safe bet. Sure, it will cost you a quarter, but twenty-five cents is cheap compared to the headache of illegal charges and identity theft . . .

Study the lay of the land. Sure, modesty might tell you to take a locker in a back section where no one can see you changing, but nobody will spot that burglar jimmying your padlock, either. Better to use a locker near the entrance; it's a much less appetizing target.

Lastly, be surreptitious about stashing anything of value in your locker, and be aware of the people around you, especially if they seem interested. If a pair of unsavory-looking characters is lurking around, or someone sits there for twenty minutes pretending to put on deodorant, you might want to reconsider. Notifying the manager is a good idea, too. The apathy of management is based on their frustration at being unable to do anything about it. Many will jump at the chance for some payback.

Stay alert and stay safe. Don't be ashamed to assume the worst about someone. If your instincts tell you something seems amiss they're probably right.

Remember: "It's not paranoia if they're really out to get you!"

HAZMAT SUIT, ANYONE?

The second most common complaint when it comes to locker room facilities – cleanliness. Two things are needed to create an unsanitary locker room: actions by members – deliberately or unintentional – and a lack of proportional effort by the gym's cleaning crew.

The Caveat Sports club in Brooklyn was a notable exception. When visiting the men's locker room during a torrential downpour, I made the remarkable discovery that its locker rooms were level with the outside sewer system. In fact, their drains were somehow interconnected. As a result, every time the sewers outside overflowed, they backed up – *into the locker room*.

It was quite a spectacle. I watched people with nose plugs trying to unpack their lockers, all the while wading through six inches of not-very-pleasant-smelling brown water.

Usually, though, the locker room attendants are blamed. This is justifiable; most of the time it's their fault.

Theirs and the company they work for.

When it comes to cleaning up after hundreds of members, lazy ain't gonna cut it. Keeping a locker room spic and span is hard, grueling work. The tiles must be scrubbed, disinfected, and hosed down – so must the showers, steam, sauna, and toilets. Then there's picking up the trash, the vacuuming, keeping the sinks clean and flowing, and washing the insides and tops of lockers. It's a lot of work. And most housekeepers that I worked with were not willingly up to the task.

Why? Consider the company that hires such people in the first place. In gyms, as in the rest of life, you get what you pay for.

Remember: minimum wage = minimal effort.

Beyond that, many of the places I worked for deliberately cut back on housekeeping hours. Sometimes, this took place on our "downtimes," i.e., the slower portions of a weekday. But sometimes it was primetime, like on a Friday afternoon from four p.m. until closing.

To me, this made absolutely no sense. The suits upstairs obviously had no idea how much damage their members could do in eight hours. And the poor staff that showed up the following morning started their shift with a nightmare on their hands (clogged sinks and toilets, and piles of trash and dirty towels) – and a mob of irate members on top of it.

I can only think of one reason for this corporate cutback: money. The way I calculate it, if you pay your housekeepers $7.00 per hour, and you cut out one eight hour shift per week, that's another $50.00+ you can keep in the company coffers (or put in your pocket). It may not sound like much, but if you multiply that number by two housekeepers per club (men's and women's, respectively), then multiply that number by, say, the 100 clubs in your chain . . . suddenly you're looking at an extra ten grand per week. That's over a half million a year. And some chains have two or three times that many locations.

Someone's really "cleaning up" out there . . .

GUILTY AS CHARGED

As easy as it is to point the finger at gym-cleaning crews, the members bear some responsibility as well. Especially when they deliberately cause the problems.

I've learned via direct observation that some male members treat their gyms like dirt – the locker room areas in particular. I can't say why this happens, but it's true. Angry clients will break locker doors, spit on the floors, and leave empty bottles and trash all over. At gyms where we gave out free towels, they'd leave soggy hair, urine, and even semen-laced towels everywhere. No joke. If a trash bin was five feet away, they'd pile their towels *around* the can instead of *in* it.

Maybe this was how they lived at home. Maybe their wives keep them on a tight leash and they took out their frustrations at the gym because it was the only place they could be slobs. Or perhaps it was their way of expressing themselves.

Some of them did far worse things.

Plumbing problems abound in gyms, and club toilets are used – and abused. It comes with the territory. I've seen stalls so scary you'd wish you had the power to levitate, but plumbing problems aren't deliberate. What *is* deliberate is when members intentionally relieve themselves outside of a stall. Showers have been graced with fecal matter in every gym I've worked for. Sometimes this is an accident. Sometimes it's a side effect of two gay guys getting it on (more on that to come). And sometimes it's a disgruntled member's way of "retaliating" against the club.

When I was a manager at Caveat Sports we had a guy who used to forgo toilet paper. He wiped himself with towels instead and left them inside stalls for fellow members to find. Infuriated clients posted signs, asking people to ID the perpetrator, so they could "catch and beat the shit out of him" (that's a direct quote).

If that wasn't bad enough, at Empirical Sports, a guy took a dump on an office chair and stashed it in the cleaning supply closet for housekeeping to find. If he thought I'd make my cleaning team deal with his little joke, he was mistaken. I had them throw a big contractor bag over the chair and toss the damned thing in the dumpster.

Needless to say, there were plenty of days when I got off work and wanted to run to the nearest ER for a tetanus shot – with some heavy duty antibiotics thrown in for good measure.

SURVIVAL TIP #14

Despite any and all efforts, health club locker rooms are, by their very nature, unsanitary. Think about it: the steam room, sauna, and showers are used by hundreds of strangers each day. Not only do people urinate in them, women change their tampons there and shove sanitary napkins down the drains, too. It's like the restroom in a gas station. Would you sit on one of their toilets?

The tiled floors in any locker room, no matter how clean they may appear, are like Petri dishes – breeding grounds for all sorts of bacterial horrors. Do yourself a favor: when you walk around your club's locker room, and most especially when you shower, do not go barefoot. Wear flip-flops, sandals, or rubber-band zip-loc bags to your feet. I don't care, but for God's sake wear something!

I caught the nastiest foot fungus imaginable from a health club shower, and it was a six month nightmare getting rid of it. Once something like that gets under the nail bed, over-the-counter remedies do nothing. It takes a liver-straining cycle of Lamisil to kill it (or, you can sit back and watch as your toes turn into hooves).

GARDEN OF HEDON

Some things that contribute to a locker room's degradation are more on the "aesthetic" side. A pet peeve of mine – one I received hundreds of complaints about over the years – is guys that, for some reason, love being naked. I've seen them in every locker room I toured, prancing around, strutting their stuff like they were in a beauty pageant.

I understand: it's a locker room – people change their clothes there. That's normal. I just can't comprehend how someone won't bother putting a change of clothes on, or anything else, for that matter. Not even a towel. They just walk around, letting it all hang out, and talk to everyone, as if all the other inhabitants of the locker room are supposed to be equally comfortable with their *au naturel* state.

Maybe they think it's a nudist colony . . .

Another thing I used to hear complaints about – guys who obsessively shave. They do it anywhere they please. Many times I opened the steam room door to find a guy with more body hair than a Labrador retriever, lathered head to toe with shaving cream, a clogged Gillette in hand. But the crème de la crème: a member told me that he was facing the mirror, trying to brush his teeth, when some "naked Neanderthal" hovered over the basin next to him, "resting one foot on top of the sink and hoisting his scrotum up so he could shave beneath his balls."

Again, that's a direct quote.

CHARACTER SPOTLIGHT: THE BALL GRABBER

Speaking of balls . . .

One afternoon, at Empirical Sports, I was sitting on a bench in the men's locker room, recovering from an intense boxing session. As I glanced across the room, I spotted a muscular male member loitering around.

Let's call this guy "Stan."

As I watched, Stan walked up to "Arnold," the men's locker room attendant. He said, "Hi," then leaned over and cupped Arnold's package. And didn't let go. Arnold was wearing a warm-up suit at the time. Unfortunately, the material clings rather nicely, so his genitals were outlined in full detail as they rested in Stan's meaty paw.

As I gaped in disbelief, Arnold, unfazed by his manhood being held captive by another man, grinned at me and chuckled. "Would you *look* at this fucking guy?"

I shook my head in disbelief. "Him? *You're* the one just standing there letting him *do* it!"

Apparently, Stan was put off by my sensitivity and wanted to initiate me into their members-only club. He released Arnold's package and started toward me. I stared at him as he smirked and extended his hand toward my crotch.

I held up one of my sweaty sneakers.

"Try it," I snarled. "And I will *feed* you this shoe."

Stan's eyes bored into mine, gauging my commitment. A second later, he retracted his hand and walked away.

Some people really need to "get a grip"...

SIGHTS BETTER LEFT UNSEEN

After misadventures like that last one, I dreaded going into health club men's rooms, particularly during a tour. It was always a crap shoot whether my clients would be enamored with the place or run screaming. I used to say a prayer before walking them in: "*Oh dear Lord, don't be mean. Please, just let the place be clean...*"

My all-time favorite locker room calamity is "the Jock Incident." I'd just signed up two college football players – big, strapping athletes who loved working out and joined without trepidation.

As I finished their paperwork and prepared to send them on their way, one of the guys pointed out that I'd forgotten to show them the locker room. Nothing could have been further from the truth; I just didn't want to risk bringing them down there. While giving a tour just the day before, I encountered this little old man. As I looked down, I noticed a huge, fleshy thing hanging between his legs. At first, I thought he was an AARP porno star, but my eyes told me otherwise. The guy had some sort of descended testicle condition; what I was looking at was his sack. Knobby and misshapen, it hung down a full twelve inches.

With that horrifying image fresh in my mind, I brushed off their request for a tour with a simple, "Bah, you've seen one locker room, you've seen 'em all."

Unfortunately, they weren't having it. They figured my locker room was just as nice as the rest of my club and I was just being lazy.

I hemmed and hawed. "C'mon, there are a lot of naked guys down there..."

"So what?" the nearest one quipped. "We're jocks. We're in locker rooms every day. Believe me, we've seen it all."

I knew he was wrong, but they left me with no alternative. I took a deep breath and brought them downstairs.

Our timing couldn't have been worse. As we walked in the door, to the right stood "Elmo," vigorously flossing a towel between his legs. Elmo was a limo driver who didn't get a lot of exercise. He weighed over 500 lbs, so you can imagine the mammoth visual we were being treated to.

Elmo spotted the looks of horror on our faces. He flushed and turned his back to us, assuming his penis was showing. Not that we could actually see it; it was swallowed up by all the fat.

Regardless, he turned away and treated us to the sight of his butts. And when I say butts, I mean plural.

There were *three* of them.

Although he had just one crack, he had three sets of cheeks, symmetrically stacked, one atop the other.

I stiffened and turned in the opposite direction, desperate to spare my clients any additional discomfort. As I swung to the left, I got no respite. Coming out of the steam room was "Gary." Gary was big. Not as big as Elmo, but at six foot two, he weighed in at 350, which is still pretty hefty. He had thick, gelatinous folds of fat that hung down like awnings over his breasts, waist, and hips. He reminded me of "Jabba the Hutt," but with an added bonus. With the exception of his bald head, Gary was covered with a layer of long, stringy body hair that made him look like a pale, overweight chimpanzee.

He waddled toward us, matted hair plastered against glistening folds of man-flesh, everything jiggling like jam.

I was sure I'd just lost my easiest sales all month. My knees locked up; I walked stiffly out the door. I stopped and stared dejectedly at the floor, waiting for my guys to tell me they were canceling. One of them put a hand on my shoulder. He took a deep breath and told me in a calm voice, "You know, Max . . . you were right. There are certain things in this life I'm just not meant to see. And that was *two* of them. We'll change in our car!"

Praise the Lord.

RIDING THE LIGHTNING

No chapter dealing with health club locker room issues would be complete without touching on steam rooms and saunas. Let me say up front, we're not talking about sex, although that is an all-too-common problem (one that we'll investigate in an upcoming chapter).

Cleanliness is, once again, the biggest issue when it comes to hot and moist environments – and abuse of the equipment itself. If improperly maintained, steams and saunas become veritable cesspools. Clients often deliberately urinate in them, leaving them stinking like a sewer. It's bad enough dealing with sweat and bacteria, but people relieving themselves there doesn't help anyone.

More industrious clients will dump water directly onto the heating elements of the sauna to increase the temperature. Sure, the red-hot coils noisily burn up the H2O and create a momentary heat blast, but that's not what they're designed to do; in fact, it's dangerous. I explained this to clients over and over again – the sauna has dry heat and the steam room moist. If they wanted the effects of the steam room they should just go in there. Trying to convert a sauna from dry to wet heat is a recipe for disaster.

They wouldn't listen.

One day at Empirical Sports, the inevitable happened. A member covered up the heating elements of the sauna with wet towels, turning it into a makeshift steam room. Once he was satisfied with his sweat, he got up and left – without removing his towels. They promptly dried out and caught fire; seconds later flames soared up the wooden walls of the place. The next thing I knew, New York's Bravest were there with hoses and axes, tearing my entire sauna apart.

Boy was I steamed.

Shortly after it was rebuilt, I caught one of my members in the act. He was more ingenious than the rest, or maybe just lazier. He used a water bottle with a nipple on the end, and whenever he wanted some more steam, he'd point the bottle at the coils and squeeze. The moment I saw the thick stream of water hit, I knew what was going on and burst in on him. I read him the riot act and also warned him of the risks.

You shouldn't play around with electricity.

I could tell from "Waterboy's" snotty attitude that he wasn't going to listen. So I told my men's locker room attendant to keep an eye on him, intending to revoke his membership if he repeated his crime.

It wasn't necessary.

Fifteen minutes later, I got an emergency call from the locker room. I rushed there to find Waterboy lying on the sauna floor. His shorts were pulled partly down, and though half-conscious, he was obviously in agony. Strong odors of ozone, urine, and burning hair filled the room. Whether he was too lazy to refill his bottle, or simply wanted to thumb his nose at me after I castigated him, he'd decided to piss on the sauna's heating elements. The powerful 220 volt current ran right back up his stream and . . . POW!

I held back my laughter until after the guy left in an ambulance. Later, I thought over the incident, and decided that I felt bad for poor Waterboy. After all, he was just trying to "spark" up his life, you know? So I called the hospital later that evening, to ask him "watts" up, and to tell him we were "positive" we weren't going to "charge" him for what he did. I even asked how much it "hertz" down there...

You don't have to say it. I know what you're thinking.

My lack of compassion is shocking.

CHAPTER 12:

HARD TO MANAGE

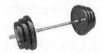

I worked as an Assistant Manager at Caveat Sports for eighteen months. During that time, I made quite a name for myself – consistently hitting big numbers for the company and making myself some decent money along the way. I learned a lot about selling, and I also discovered things about my employers that I wasn't exactly thrilled with. Still, I had few complaints; I had a great social life, and the job was entertaining.

One complaint I *did* have was my current Area Manager, "Danny." Danny had replaced Johnson. He and I weren't exactly the best of friends. In fact, I disliked him intensely. He enjoyed abusing his power. For example, he used to kidnap whichever of my receptionists he was hot for at the moment (so she could help him outside with his "administrative duties"), while leaving me with an unmanned front desk.

Eventually, Danny's abuse of his authority came back to bite him on the ass. One day, he sent me on a seventy-mile trek to do some risqué shopping for him. I was hardly enthusiastic about it; I'd just gotten my driver's license and didn't even own a car. Danny ignored my protestations. He made me take his rental and laughed about how I'd miss out on sales (which he'd gladly pocket in my absence).

As karma would have it, while driving on the highway, the driver ahead of me unexpectedly slammed on his breaks. After reaching for the radio, I looked up to see five car lengths rapidly becoming one. I put the brake pedal through the floor before crashing violently into the next vehicle. The impact was horrendous, and if it weren't for my seatbelt, I'd have flown right through the windshield.

I sat there, stunned and disoriented, and gradually realized I'd just destroyed my boss's car. Ninety minutes later, I drove the smoking hulk back to my club. Danny freaked. It turned out the rental was in his name only, and his insurance wouldn't cover the accident. Worse, I'd filed a police report. He ended up taking the car to his cousin's collision shop, costing him seven grand – which he claimed was half what the rental company would have charged him. Being a "nice guy," he said he expected me to pay only half, since it was his decision to send me on the trip.

I never gave him a dime, and he never brought it up to me again.

So, I was more than a little surprised when I got a call from Danny several months later, offering me a promotion to General Manager. I was intrigued. Being a GM would mean a substantial increase in pay, and I'd be running an entire club. The only downside was that the club he had in mind was in the city, which meant a forty-minute train ride to work. Sure, that's a standard commute for most people, but I had a cozy little apartment only three blocks from my current club, so for me it was a major inconvenience.

I thought over Danny's offer, weighing the pros and cons. I knew that this type of promotion usually occurs after a manager is fired and someone is needed to fill the gap. It would be a high-pressure position, with long hours and the club's entire quota resting on my shoulders. Before he was fired, my previous manager joked that being a boss for Caveat Sports meant putting your head on a high-speed escalator that led straight to the corporate chopping block. You're responsible for everything – and if something goes wrong, it lands like a guillotine, squarely on the GM's neck.

Despite these misgivings, I accepted Danny's offer. Within ten minutes I'd packed my bags and was headed into the city.

NO MAN'S LAND

To my surprise, I discovered that my new club was a small, women's-only facility. Oh, the *irony*.

Now, you'd *think* that a horny toad like me would be in paradise, but you'd be wrong. Don't get me wrong, there were lots of attractive females there, but I could tell right away that most of my clientele didn't want men anywhere near them. They were either:

1) Really hot model-types who didn't want to be bothered.
2) Unattractive, overweight women I wouldn't *want* to bother, or:

3) Man-hating lesbians who viewed me as competition, and whom I'd
   better not bother.

However, I quickly realized that I had bigger problems than that – the
club I'd inherited was a nightmare.

The entire place was barely bigger than my apartment. It had a tiny
aerobics studio, bordered by a fitness area comprised of six weight machines and eight pieces of cardio – and that was it. During the day, the place
was empty. There was a small lunch hour crowd, but at 5 p.m. "the herd" descended like a stampede from an old-fashioned western. I had hundreds of
girls packed like cordwood. Crowds lined up, twelve-chicks-deep, for every
weight and cardio machine. The jammed classes overflowed the aerobics
floor and spilled onto the adjacent gym area.

Members waited for an hour just to do a few lousy sets, while all around
them people wove in and out and jumped up and down. Collisions were
non-stop, arguments were constant, and the threat of injury and lawsuits
loomed over the place like a malevolent cloud. The air conditioning was
barely adequate to begin with – throw in all those hot, sweaty bodies in
such close quarters, and my club became the world's funkiest sauna.

PORT IN A STORM

I learned very quickly not to venture onto the gym floor at rush hour. As
crowded as the place was when I got there, my aggressive selling tactics
made matters worse. A few weeks after taking the helm, I was cornered by
a group of infuriated hellions who'd deduced that I was responsible for jamming the club to the point of bursting.

They were correct, of course.

They wanted my head – or at least my testicles – and *not* in a good way.
When they told me they would contact my superiors and complain about
me signing up too many people, I tried not to laugh. If anything, that'd get
me a commendation.

On a positive note, as hot and steamy as my club was during peak hours
(the term "rain forest" was frequently tossed around), my office had its own,
separate AC vent. If I kept my door closed, it stayed nice and cool. It was a
sanctuary for me and my co-workers, and also made closing sales much easier. Keeping my door closed also shielded me from disgruntled members, of
which there were plenty. I could hear them giving my receptionists a hard
time through the office walls.

Better them than me!

Editor's Note: in order to sell under these conditions, the trick was to talk even louder than the angry members complaining outside. By drowning them out, my soon-to-be clients never realized what awaited them . . .

BRING IT ON!

Occasionally, arguments escalated into actual fistfights. To prevent total anarchy, Caveat Sports clubs have sign-up sheets at the front desk for their cardio machines, usually with thirty-minute time limits. And the rules are strict. There's no calling in for reservations, no signing, leaving, and coming back. This setup tends to keep conflicts to a minimum.

Note the phrase: *"tends* to". . .

It was around 4:30 p.m. – a good half-hour before the deluge. The place was busy, but survivable. Winding my way through the cardio machines, I saw two women, a well-built brunette and a sultry-looking blonde, screaming at one another over a treadmill. Apparently, the first woman took too long to wipe down her machine, costing her successor a few precious minutes.

As I drew closer, their words became more heated. They started pushing and shoving; a second later, it became an all-out brawl.

I leapt between them and pulled them apart; they were like two crazed alley cats. As I tried to play peacemaker, I noticed them eyeing me up and down. They exchanged angry-but-conspiratorial glances, then focused on me. I didn't need ESP to know what was going through their heads.

"Let's kill him first, and then settle this between ourselves."

A heartbeat later, they flew at me like demons. Suddenly, I was blocking a barrage of punches and kicks, with the majority meant for my more vulnerable regions. I backed away, cursing angrily, and went to call the police.

Let *them* handle it. At least they got combat pay.

STANDING ROOM ONLY

Regardless of your martial arts skills, crowded conditions and lack of available equipment can be problematic at even the priciest places. That's because most health clubs have huge membership bases, with some hosting 20,000+ clients.

As a manager, one of the first things I learned is that most of those people never go. They're the ideal clients – they pay for nothing. Even so, most gyms at rush hour are like Manhattan trains: jammed to the gills with tired, sweaty sardines.

SURVIVAL TIP #15

Aerobics classes can also be a problem at crowded clubs. It should raise a big, red flag if the studio you're touring has numbers labeled (or worse, spray painted) on the floor. They're there to make sure no riots break out.

Also, before you join a gym, find out what their class policy is. Besides a fee, are you required to reserve a spot in the boxing and spinning classes? How far in advance can you reserve? And is there some "old boy" network in place where members with seniority always get their names on the list with no problem, whereas new people who call the minute the club opens can never get a spot?

All, questions well worth having answered before your trial period ends.

COLD HEARTED

Besides the overcrowded conditions and poor ventilation, my gym also suffered from a major cleanliness problem. There were simply too many resentful members occupying too small an area.

As if to worsen things, the corporate office suddenly decided to cut back on my housekeeping hours. Because it was relatively quiet during the day and nearly dead after 8 p.m., they decided that only the 12-8:00 shift was necessary.

It was a bad move. The amount of damage being done up until eight was staggering, and it continued until close to nine, when the last stragglers finally called it a night. The one housekeeper did the best she could, but there was no way she could get to everything. Overtime was a big no-no with my company. Worst of all, everything that took place after eight was left completely untouched for the members who came in the following morning, who started their day with the sight of a filthy locker room.

I went to Danny, figuring he'd help. He told me in no uncertain terms that I had the maximum allowance of housekeeping hours for my club, and there would be no more forthcoming. When I pointed out the dismal conditions of my club, that it was upsetting the clients and even affecting sales, he suggested I stay for an extra couple hours – after my twelve-hour shift – and mop and scrub the place myself.

Danny was rapidly proving himself to be an impediment – maybe he was still angry about the car crash. One day, though, he showed me a malicious side of himself that went far beyond just holding a grudge. I'd just signed up a young woman who was a recovering rape victim. A burglar had come through her window in the middle of the night and held a knife to her throat while he sexually assaulted and sodomized her. As a result, she came to my gym because she was (understandably) afraid to train around men.

I have sisters, so naturally I felt very bad for her. But when I told Danny about my client, figuring he'd sympathize with her horrific ordeal, he chuckled and made a sadistic joke that she probably sat alone by her window every night, pining for the rapist to return so he could have his way with her again.

OUT OF THE FRYING PAN

Despite everything that was stacked against me, I focused on making the best of my situation and eventually found a groove. Once I figured out the best times to go onto the gym floor (and when to avoid it), I could resume my omnipresent sexual addiction.

And there was an added bonus. My previous health club had been in a predominantly Italian and Russian neighborhood. This meant that the majority of the women I encountered (and dated) were of those nationalities. That was fine and dandy at the time, but variety is the spice of life.

The city clubs, by their very locale, offered a far more diverse gene pool to immerse myself in, and I quickly found myself romantically involved with women from all parts of the globe. I was in paradise.

Unfortunately, my Garden of Eden had a few serpents slithering around it.

For the first time in my career, I was having problems hitting my numbers – and my superiors weren't happy about it. When you're the manager of a health club, your quotas and budgets are your primary concern. You may work in a "service industry," but the well-being of your members runs a very distant second. The bosses want money, pure and simple. And they're relying on you to get it for them. If you fail, they'll very quickly find someone else.

The problem was that my trial-period cancelations were phenomenally high. In the case of a Caveat Sports membership, and for most other facilities, clients have a three-day money-back guarantee.

When I first took over the club, my predecessor gave me some sage advice before cleaning out his desk. This consisted of tips on how to overcome clients' complaints about the size of the club, by pitching women on the sanctity of having their own, male-free environment, regardless of how small.

He also taught me his secret to success: screwing people over so they couldn't cancel. He never allowed new clientele to be exposed to the horrors of his club until after their trial period had passed. He did so by informing them that – for safety's sake – they couldn't use the place until after their complimentary personal training session. Coincidentally, their appointment with said trainer ended up being a solid *four* business days after they joined. By the time they came in to train – and screamed in horror at what they found – it was already too late to do anything about it. They were stuck paying for the next three years, whether they used the place or not.

Unfortunately, narcissistic creature that I was, I still had some scruples. And no matter how much my club needed sales, I couldn't bring myself to call upon my predecessor's "delaying tactic" to screw people over like that.

My crisis of conscience would prove costly . . .

DRUNK WITH POWER

Since I was unwilling to deceive clients into three-year contracts, the cancelation rate soon reached a frightening 30%. As a case study, it showed how consumers will react to a poorly maintained health club if they know their cancelation rights.

On the downside, I was unable to hit my club's quota.

It didn't matter how hard I and my team worked. In our eyes, we "hit" each and every month. Sometimes we even went 10-15% over our numbers (an astonishing feat, considering our club was the size of a broom closet). But when our members saw the awful conditions they'd be dealing with, the three-day cancels came piling in. Even 115% eventually came crashing back down to a mere 85% of budget.

My inability to hit started affecting me financially. All of a sudden, I wasn't getting those juicy bonuses, which form much of a manager's income. I was working 9 a.m. to 9 p.m., Monday to Friday. That meant I was putting in at least 60 hours per week; yet despite the extra fifteen hours, plus ten hours per week in traveling time, I was barely making the same money I did back when I was an Assistant Manager.

I had a much bigger problem that that, though: "Jack Daniels."

I'm not talking about the liquor. Jack was Danny's immediate superior – a Regional Director who ran scores of clubs with an iron fist. I call him JD because, according to rumor, he was a big-time alcoholic. At first I didn't know whether that was true. I did observe Jack sitting at a big table during monthly meetings, pouring himself glass after glass from a large pitcher of some dark beverage that looked suspiciously like rum and coke. I also overheard Danny talking to him on speakerphone. Unaware that he was being taped, Jack screamed at Danny in what was obviously a drunken rage, spouting every profanity in the book.

And this was in the early afternoon.

In my eyes, Jack was the stereotypical example of absolute power corrupting absolutely. He was well dressed and charismatic, and used that and his position to his advantage. He liked to travel around to his assorted clubs, and when he found an attractive, young woman "working under him," he immediately took her under his wing. He'd pull her out of her club, promoting her so that she answered to him and him alone. One of these women was a lowly receptionist. He yanked her out of her gym and, within two weeks, made her a full-fledged manager. She went from making minimum wage to $80K+ per year overnight.

Jack was very possessive when it came to his women, and quite willing to abuse his power to both land and keep them. Back when I was a personal trainer, I worked alongside a sales rep named "Luke" who was romantically interested in my current manager. She liked Luke as well, and had not yet succumbed to any of Jack's offers. When Jack found out about his "competition" he utilized an expeditious-but-petty way to fire the hapless guy. He called the club and ordered Luke placed at the front desk to answer the phones. He then called over and over, and each time the guy answered, Jack would wait a few seconds, then hang up in his face.

Inevitably, Luke grew weary of being hung up on – not to mention the monotony of repeating the same, boring company greeting. His temper finally got the better of him. I was standing there when it happened. The phone rang for the umpteenth time, and he picked it up and said, "Look, jerk-off, why don't you just call somewhere else for a change?"

Of course, it was Jack Daniels on the line. Jack pretended it was his first call and went completely ape, firing Luke on the spot for inappropriate language and answering the phone in an unprofessional manner.

When it came to the girls Jack "cultivated," there were many rumors of what he got in return for their meteoric rises. I can't vouch for any of this personally, but based on the body language of the women he surrounded himself with, coupled with reports I got from women he promoted and then tried becoming intimate with, I'm sure he got his fair share of job perks.

One should never be surprised what people will do for money. Or that an avaricious woman would allow a man like Jack to "liquor."

THE BREAKING POINT

Speaking of money, once it became apparent my club was having a problem hitting, I started getting phone calls from Jack. And I don't mean encouraging, pat-on-the-back, "you can do it" type pep talks. They were barrages of vile threats from the slurred lips of a raging alky on the mother of all benders. He used to call me up, curse me out, insult me, scream at me, and threaten my job, all in one tequila-laced breath. It didn't matter to him that I was doing better than any other manager in the city; it wasn't good enough.

Even without the added fear of being fired, my finances were on shaky ground. I got so stressed out from Jack's ongoing abuse that, when I ran my fingers through my hair (to keep from screaming), a hundred hairs fell out. And the men in my family don't lose their hair.

One night, I awoke in the middle of a terrifying nightmare. A giant squid was trying to eat me. When I opened my eyes, I could still see its tentacles, writhing like snakes as they wormed their way into my bedroom.

Things were getting bad. And I mean *real* bad. You can only subject people to so much duress before something finally gives. Either they cry for their mother and run away, or they snap.

I've never been much of a runner.

I started having the most awful dream. I would drive to my family's home in Pennsylvania, pick up my rifle and shotgun, and then drive back to my company's monthly sales meeting. When I got there, everyone was already seated inside the fancy meeting hall. With lengths of chain, I proceeded to quickly and quietly lock all the exit doors from the outside – all except one. Then I threw open that remaining door and walked briskly into the meeting. Before the confused gazes of everyone present, I locked the last exit from the inside, then smiled and chambered a round into my trusty 12-gauge.

I guess you can figure out what happened next . . .

I started having this dream repeatedly, and not just when I was asleep. If I sat at my desk and let my mind wander, it came to me. Worst of all, I was beginning to enjoy it. I found myself relishing the imagined looks of terror on the faces of those who mistreated me.

I know I sound like someone who was headed for a nice stretch in Bellevue. But I truly believe if something hadn't happened to break the cycle of cruelty, it's possible I'd have reached a breaking point and made that dream a reality.

Jack and his cronies had no idea how close they might have come.

Fortunately for everyone, I caught a break. Out of nowhere, I was transferred out of my club to a nearby location. Unfortunately, the poor girl who replaced me as manager did even worse than I did, and was subjected to the same mistreatment, if not worse. She became so desperate she resorted to calling me at my club, usually hysterical. In between sobs, she pleaded with me to give her advice on how to build her business and cope with the abuse she was getting from higher up.

I gave her whatever pointers I could, both for generating sales and holding onto business. I also tried to bolster her spirits, telling her any jokes I knew to cheer her up, while trying to convince her she was strong enough to handle whatever tortures they were piling on her.

She wasn't. A few months later, she suffered a cerebral aneurysm and died.

That's right: *died*.

And this girl was an athletic thirty-year-old who used to run *marathons*.

Apparently the company didn't want anyone talking about her dying. I was told by my supervisor that no one was allowed to discuss her – and that anyone who did would be fired. I don't know what their agenda was; maybe they were worried about bad press or a wrongful death suit. In the end, though, they could say whatever they wanted. I know what they subjected people to because I went through it myself.

And I believe they stressed that poor girl to death.

ABSOLUTELY PRICELESS: HOW TO BEAT YOUR STAFF

Not all health club higher-ups are satisfied with just inflicting verbal or psychological abuse on their underlings. Some of them like to take a more "hands-on" approach when it comes to keeping their team in line. I've seen numerous managers restrained by staff members who, otherwise, would have viciously attacked their employees. I have also been personally threatened with violence by my superiors, and offered to bring bodily harm to another, in turn.

In fitness, violence in the workplace is fairly common. Much more so than people would think, or the gym owners would like you to believe.

A few months after I'd been transferred to my Caveat Sports in the city, I swung by my old club in Brooklyn. I was on my way home and figured I'd say hello to my colleague "Apollo," the club's current manager.

When I walked in his office, Apollo was holding court with his Assistant Manager "Bag" and his head trainer "Extra." From what I could see, Bag was acting rebellious about something that his boss was pressuring him to do.

As I stood in the doorway, with Extra to my right, Apollo and Bag suddenly started roughhousing and "slap-boxing" (where you pretend-spar and lightly tap your opponent with your fingertips instead of actually punching them).

Slap-boxing is not the smartest of sports. Two grown men can't smack each other in the face, no matter how lightly, for very long without their testosterone levels surging out of control. I've seen many a slap-boxing match escalate into an actual fight, but never so quickly. One second they were standing there, smirking and jibing one another, and the next I heard Apollo say, "Oh, you wanna *do* this? Let's *do* this!"

A second later, he pulled Bag's shirt up and over his head, blinding him, and started barraging him with full power hooks and uppercuts.

It took a moment for me to realize that the General Manager of one of our health clubs was pummeling a subordinate right in front of me, and with members walking back and forth outside his office. I glanced at Extra, indicating that we should intervene, only to have him stare confusedly at me.

"Don't just stand there!" I yelled.

I plunged into the fray, forcibly pulling a furious Apollo off his victim and restraining him in a full nelson.

With Extra's help, Bag managed to get to his feet, but he had to lean against a nearby wall for support. He'd definitely gotten the worst of it. He was dazed, bleeding from his nose and mouth, and he staggered outside to clear his head.

Inside, Apollo stalked back in forth like a caged lion, cursing and going on and on about how he was going to "beat his assistant's ass."

Ever the peacemaker, I calmed Apollo down, then went outside and did the same for Bag. I even managed to have them shake hands before I left, which was a good thing for Apollo. He was lucky I liked him. If I hadn't, I'd have told Bag to call 911 and then collapse on the sidewalk. Apollo would've been arrested for assault and battery and fired. And Bag would've ended up with a huge lawsuit against the company. The poor kid was brutalized by his own boss, and with eyewitnesses to prove it.

Oh well. Once beaten, twice shy . . .

SURVIVAL TIP #16

This one is for anyone working in fitness. If you're considering a job with one of the larger chains, be prepared to deal with characters like the ones I just mentioned. And if you want to survive more than a month or two, take this advice to heart: Be Switzerland. Be friendly with everyone, say nothing bad about anyone, and pretend you like everybody, no matter how mean or treacherous they may seem.

Health clubs are filled to the ceiling with frustrated individuals whose sole existence revolves around gossiping. Anything bad you say about someone, even jokingly, will make it back to that person, and you will find yourself with an enemy. Make enough enemies, and eventually someone in a position of power will find an opportunity to destroy you.

Far better to play it safe and kiss every ass you can. That way, should an irate member file a complaint against you (for whatever reason), you'll have a crowd of people waiting to defend you, instead of an eager assassin, sharpening the blade they've been waiting to bury in your back.

ABSOLUTELY PRICELESS: THE CHICKEN MAN

When it comes to handling job stress, some managers deal differently than others. I knew one who used to sneak out for a three-martini lunch, another who (under the guise of "prospecting") would creep out for a quick bootie call, and still another who simply went out to his car, rolled up a fat joint, and smoked his way back to sanity.

When I worked at Empirical Sports, my manager, "Sal," exhibited a truly unique way of dealing with stress. I knew he was having a hard time. He told me the Area Manager who convinced him to move to New York and take the job was "full of shit" (direct quote). He said she'd lied to him about every aspect of the job, from compensation on up.

What I didn't know was that Sal was reaching his breaking point.

One afternoon, I walked out of my office, a contract in hand. I heard a loud scream, and turned to see Sal slam down his phone and lunge to his feet. His face was a mask of unfettered exasperation as he cleared his desk with wide sweeps of his arms. His computer monitor, keyboard, pens, stapler, contract bins – all went crashing to the floor.

Not used to such outbursts, or Sal's destructive behavior, I stared transfixed.

Before my eyes, he climbed onto his desk . . .

Editor's Note: Back in college, I had the misfortune of finding a classmate who'd committed suicide by hanging himself. It was not a good experience – especially since I came face to face with him in the dark, after he'd been hanging for two days in 90-degree heat.

With that image lurking in the back of my mind, my immediate fear was that I was about to watch Sal attempt to kill himself. I looked fearfully upward, but to my relief saw no rope.

A second later, Sal turned into a six-foot chicken, right before my eyes.

His gangly-limbed impersonation was spot-on, and came complete with head bobs and clucks, his loafers scratching repeatedly at the ground as he dug for feed. For a full minute he remained there, flapping away and belting out a chorus of "cock-a-doodle-doos," while a parade of startled members walked back and forth.

We're talking about a conservative, forty year-old man, wearing a shirt and tie, and working in a corporate environment.

At a loss how to proceed in the face of this insanity, I mumbled a low, *"Okay . . ."* and retreated to the safety of my office.

After a few minutes of this, Sal stopped. He climbed nimbly down from his perch and proceeded to pick everything up off the floor, putting it carefully back on his desk and arranging it exactly as before. Then, once his desk was properly organized, he sat down in his chair and went calmly back to work. I could see the look on his face, and it was as if nothing out of the ordinary had transpired

I didn't say anything.

Not surprisingly, Sal quit the company shortly thereafter. A few months later, I brought up the "chicken man" incident to "Caesar," the next Area

Manager who took over our district. When I gave him the details of my story, Caesar became very agitated. He warned me quite sternly that I was to never, *ever* repeat what I'd seen. Not to anyone, under any circumstances.

To be honest, I wasn't too keen about Caesar's blatantly authoritarian style of managing, or his "directive."

But hey – no harm, no fowl . . .

CHAPTER 13:

(NOT SO) BRAVE NEW WORLD

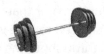

When I was unexpectedly transferred from my tiny, women's-only club, it turned out to be a mixed blessing. Although it freed me from an ongoing barrage of maltreatment (and possibly prevented me from losing my mind), Danny informed me that, due to my inexperience and the size of the new club, I'd be splitting control with another manager.

I was a little put off at first, but when I found out I would still get my full base salary, it was fine by me. Besides, it wasn't like I had any say in the matter. In addition, when the other manager turned out to be "Harry," someone I'd worked with at my first club, I was relieved. Harry and I got on well, and it would be a pleasant change working with someone I had a halfway decent relationship with.

The club itself turned out to be a bit of a disappointment. Although it was co-ed and much larger and better equipped than my previous command (including pool, Jacuzzi, steam and sauna), it was still stifling hot and crowded at peak hours. Whereas my old club had about 4,000 members, this one had closer to 12,000.

Still, the substantial increase in square footage did help. At least there were only three or four people waiting in line for weight machines at 5 p.m., as opposed to the ten or twelve I was used to.

My initial concern that Harry might view me as unwelcome competition for sales was unfounded. He was very happy to see me; in fact, he greeted me with open arms. At first I thought it was because the girl I replaced (who died shortly thereafter, God rest her soul) had been competitive or confrontational, but I was wrong. It was a comfort zone issue. Harry wanted to share leadership with someone he could trust, and he figured that someone would be me.

Of course, the "why" of it all turned out to be very amusing. As a General Manager, Harry took a lot of liberties. He loved showing up whenever he felt like it. Our shifts normally ran from 9-9:00 p.m., but I was informed by Danny that Harry often came in an hour or two late. He asked me to keep track and immediately report any tardiness on Harry's part.

Ignorant of this, and figuring with me there he didn't have to watch his back anymore, Harry grew very relaxed. Instead of showing up at 10 or 11 o'clock, he'd come strolling in at 12 noon or even 1 p.m. He justified this by saying he stayed in the club far later than normal, usually until closing, which was at midnight. He also used to take very long lunches and several twenty-minute smoke breaks throughout the day.

I had no problem with any of this. Nor did I rat Harry out to Danny – not even once. I'm not a stoolie. Besides, for me, Harry's creative scheduling was a blessing. As managers, he and I took turns in terms of who got what business. With him absent, everything that walked in the door for that first 3-4 hours, and whenever he disappeared for his nicotine fix, was fair game, and I loved it.

It was a symbiotic relationship. Once Harry realized I wasn't looking to advance myself at his expense, and that he could count on me, he was content. With me reliably holding down the fort and covering his ass, he had the freedom to do whatever it was he did around there, which sure as hell didn't seem to be making money.

When I eventually discovered how he spent a lot of his time, I was tickled pink.

DEEP THOUGHTS

Harry's sexual preference was constant topic of conversation among my coworkers. Everyone at my first club in Brooklyn was convinced he was gay. I couldn't have cared less, but if he was, I wasn't aware of it. He regularly walked around cracking "fag" jokes and acting like a typical gym stud. And there were always girls hanging out in his office. I even saw an attractive blonde walk in and do a strip tease in his lap. He seemed to enjoy it, so I assumed he was straight.

One day, though, something happened that convinced me perhaps Harry wasn't being entirely honest about his sexuality. It involved, of all things, my lunch.

Back when I was a sales rep, I had a bad habit of hitting the local hotdog stand for lunch and choking down a cola and a hot sausage. Harry used to abuse me for eating such "crap" and he was right; it was very unhealthy. But it was also fast and cheap, and I was on a tight budget.

One day, sitting with him over lunch, I told him about this gorgeous Venezuelan babe I'd hooked up with the night before. I explained that, in technical terms, she'd given me what was, without a doubt, the most amazing fellatio of my life. I recounted the experience to him in full detail, including the part where I kept screaming "Oh God!" over and over as everything around me turned gray.

I stepped out a little while later. When I came back, I found Harry sitting at his desk with not one, but *three* hot sausages piled up in front of him. I just stood there and stared. He looked up and gave me this bewildered look that basically said he had no idea *why* he was eating all those big, unhealthy tube steaks; he just couldn't help himself.

Shortly after that, Harry was promoted to manager. And right after *that*, he started hanging out after hours in the club with some of his male friends. It was then that those nasty condoms started showing up. At that point, I started to wonder about Harry – not that it was a big deal (I don't mean the condom thing. That was disgusting, pure and simple. I mean that, in this day and age, nobody ultimately cared if he was gay or not).

Regardless of what anyone said or thought, though, Harry kept up his anti-gay comments and jokes. Maybe it was because the rumors were unfounded, or maybe it was because our gym was located in a tough Italian neighborhood and he felt safer "playing it straight."

NO MORE CLOSET SPACE

Eventually, I found out that, despite all his denials, pretenses, and protestations, Harry was, in fact, completely gay. Even more ironically, I was the one that ended up "exposing him."

We were working together in the city one evening, and he decided to cut out early. It was near quitting time, and I was about to get the hell out of Dodge with two of my friends. As we headed for the door, my office phone rang. When I answered, a deep, masculine voice asked, "Is Harry there?"

"No," I said. "He left already."

"Are you sure? He said he'd be there."

"Sorry, pal. He's not here."

I hung up and jabbed a speakerphone line so I could check my answering machine. I found that the call I'd just gotten was a three-way, and the guy was still connected, along with several others. His voice however, had changed drastically, switching from the manly tone he'd used on me to a lilting, effeminate voice. I heard him say, "He said he's not there; I don't understand."

A whole group of obviously gay men chimed in, and my friends and I gaped at one other. We realized we had a rare opportunity to garner a glimpse into what was, to us, an alien world. Now *this* was entertainment! Without a word, I hit the mute button and cranked up the speakerphone. We pulled up some stools and sat there for the next fifteen minutes, listening to them talk about which among them was more of a whore, who would be whose date for an upcoming gay wedding, and so forth.

After a while, the novelty wore off. It wasn't until they started talking about Harry – who was romantically involved with one of them – that our ears pricked up again. The next few minutes became more than we could handle, and I finally pulled the plug.

I didn't say anything to Harry about the phone call – at least not at first. I was content I knew the truth and left it at that. Like I said, it wasn't that big of a deal.

Eventually, though, I was forced to come clean.

As I said, Harry had a bad habit of showing up late for work. I also noticed that when he dragged himself in, he was always stiff and hunched over, and he complained about how badly his back was "killing him" – especially, if it was a Monday. He'd stagger in to our shared office and rail about the pain he was in, using it as an excuse to steal my seat.

One day, as I watched him lower himself into the manager's chair, I remembered the call from a few months prior. Like a smack in the face, it dawned on me that it wasn't his *back* that was hurting him; it was a part of his anatomy a little farther south.

I told my theory to a coworker. That following Monday, we were sitting in my office and watched as Harry, true to form, came stumbling in. He was dragging his feet and groaning, "Oh God, my back . . . get up . . . my back is killing me!" My friend and I exchanged looks and just cracked up.

Harry's eyes flew open wide and he flipped out immediately.

"Fuck you guys!" he barked.

At this point I was tired of the pretense, and had my colleague leave the office. I confessed to Harry all about the phone call, and then told him point-blank, "Look, I *know* you're gay, and I don't *give* a damn. Okay?"

After he got over his initial trepidation about being "outed" and realized I was safe to talk to, Harry's innate nature asserted itself. He wanted to know what the guys on the phone had said about him. And I mean he *really* wanted to know. He wouldn't let up, and for a week straight just kept prodding me for info.

It just goes to show, curiosity can come back to haunt you.

Sometimes ignorance really *is* bliss.

Editor's Note: Although I knew the truth, Harry continued to keep up appearances with both our members and superiors. His efforts to conceal his obvious orientation eventually became a running joke. Once, our Area Manager asked me to check on a rarely used closet by the front desk. As I opened it, he asked me, "What's in there?" I peeked inside, made an astonished face, and exclaimed, "Harry!"

The guy laughed for a week.

ABSOLUTELY PRICELESS: IT'S MY TREAT!

I guess Harry started rubbing off on me (no pun intended), because I once used some "mildly inappropriate" language on our mutual boss that I'm sure he could've related to.

One fine day, Danny (the manager whose car I destroyed) was lurking about. My best friend and I were hiding out in my office, trying our best to avoid him. We were putting together plans for a big fishing trip, and we knew if Danny found out, he'd force us to take him. Unfortunately, he materialized in my doorway just as we were counting the cash for our deposit. He saw the money and froze, his hands gripping the edges of the doorframe.

"Hey, what's all the cash for?" he asked.

We were cornered, so I decided to go with a direct approach.

"It's the deposit for our shark-fishing trip," I replied.

"Great, count me in!"

My friend and I exchanged irritated looks. He felt the same way I did about Danny.

"Fine, $75," I said, holding out my hand.

"W-what?" Danny stammered.

I was laughing inside. I knew he was cheap, and it was the surest way to fend him off.

"You heard me," I continued. The trip is $800, and the deposit is $300. $300 divided by four is $75 each. Let's see your green."

"I'll uh . . . I'll give it to you later."

"Oh *no*. If you're going, we need commitment, so let's have the cash."

Danny fidgeted, his tiny eyes blinking. He decided to throw his weight around, figuring that would win the day.

"You guys should treat me," he announced.

I tried to not look flabbergasted. "We should *what*? Are you kidding me?"

"No. I'm very good to you guys. You should treat me."

"Let me see if I've got this straight," I said. "We bust our asses for peanuts while you pull in 100K because of our hard work, and you're telling me *we* should treat *you*?"

"Yep," he said, nodding as if it was decided.

I gave my friend a look, and then said something I'd never said to anyone.

"Sure thing, Danny." I smirked. "I'll treat you alright. I'll treat you to my asshole. *All* you can eat. It's a *buffet*!"

If he wanted corn, I'd need a day's notice.

Danny turned sheet white. His jaw dropped; he tried saying my name, but only a strangled "Duh!" came out of his mouth. A second later, his arms dropped to his sides and he staggered off like a drunk looking for a place to pass out. Meanwhile, my pal – trying desperately not to laugh – started shaking from head to toe. His bones turned to butter and he slid onto the floor. He lay there in a fetal position, hysterically cackling.

Amazingly, my boss never brought up the fact that I flat-out told him to eat my ass. It was like he went into denial. I guess it was so unfathomable to him that one of his beleaguered employees could be so rude and disrespectful that his brain just couldn't handle it. To this day, I am the only person I know of who's told something like that to their superior – and one I wasn't even on good terms with – and didn't get into trouble.

Now *that's* what I call a treat.

WELCOME TO THE JUNGLE

Speaking of feasting on rump roast . . .

It's a fairly well-known fact that steam rooms and saunas attract horny gay guys. Historically speaking, homosexual men go to places like that for quick and easy action. It's a cultural thing that's existed since the days of Roman bathhouses. Now, let me just say up front that there's nothing wrong with being gay. It's a lifestyle choice, and what people do in their private lives is their business.

That being said, let me also say that there *is* a time and a place for everything.

Just about every gym I worked at had a problem with gay men acting out their fantasies. And the gym Harry and I were running was no exception. I discovered there were two types of people who came to my gym. One came to work out, and the other came to get it on in my sauna, steam room, and bathroom stalls.

As a gym manager, having men engaging in group sex in the locker room is very bad for business; it's socially unacceptable and unsanitary. That being said, I made it a point to strictly enforce company policy: *anyone* caught performing a sexual act in my club (straight or gay) was thrown out immediately. This may seem hypocritical, given my own transgressions, but at least my crimes took place after closing. And let's face facts, those in charge – including a few of our past Presidents – don't always abide by the rules.

The problem was catching them in the act. Most guys who gather in public places to get their groove on know the consequences of their actions if they get caught. They thus tend to be organized. My problem customers would often post a spotter, known colloquially as a "chickie," to stand guard. The chickie kept watch for approaching employees and rapped on the glass when they spotted one, giving their colleagues plenty of time to clean up their act before they got busted.

With such behavior running rampant, my staff conducted organized campaigns to catch the perpetrators. It was like a warped chess match. My housekeepers managed to nail the worst offenders without any outside assistance. That was easy. Overly horny men don't tend to make the smartest decisions.

For example, one day my fitness manager noticed a member seated in one of our bathroom stalls. We could see his feet – along with a pair of large, brown paper grocery bags right in front of him. When we saw one of the paper bags move it was obvious something weird was going on. My FM kicked in the door, hitting the guy – who was standing with his feet inside the bags – in the rear end and sending him crashing into his friend's face. Judging from the startled yelp and simultaneous choking sounds, it must have been the sitter's first "deep throat" experience.

When it came to catching the more organized offenders, the other members often volunteered to help. A lot of our clients were fed up with the goings-on in their steam room and sauna, which made it impossible for them to use the facilities they were paying good money for.

One member regularly asked my housekeepers to wait around the corner from the sauna. Then he'd walk by the chickie standing guard, giving him a suggestive smile or wink. As soon as he spotted guys engaging in lewd acts, he'd whistle and the housekeeper would come running, catching the perpetrators in the act. They were then rounded up and brought to my office.

I had a "well-oiled" lecture I gave anyone caught screwing in my locker rooms. Then I cut up their membership card and sent them packing.

One of my favorites was this guy we busted giving head. I took his membership card and checked his license to make sure I had the right guy. Then I asked him if he knew why he was in my office. He said no, and played the stalling game until I had to spell it out.

"Okay, you want to be that way, fine," I said. "You were caught performing fellatio on another man in my sauna. Does that ring a bell?"

"B-but . . . it was an *accident*!" he exclaimed.

"An "accident"? Oh, I see . . . so you slipped and *fell* on his cock. Well, that explains everything!"

He stared at the floor.

"Listen . . ." I began for the umpteenth time. "I don't care what you do in your home, the backseat of a car, a movie theater, or a motel. It's none of my business. But this is a health club, and the type of behavior you exhibited will not be tolerated. Your membership is revoked. Get out, and don't ever come back."

The next day, a personal trainer named "Oscar" tried giving me lip about the aforementioned incident. Oscar was sixty and had worked at the club as a floor trainer for the past thirty years. He was also an actor.

Editor's Note: Maybe it's just me, but how talented an actor can you be if you're still working a gym floor after three decades, making only seven bucks an hour?

Oscar came barging into my office.

"I can't believe you threw 'John' out," he barked.

I cocked an eyebrow. "John? He violated club policy. Is there a problem?"

"You can't just revoke the guy's membership like that!"

"Of course I can." I gave him an annoyed look. "He was giving *head* in my sauna. He's gone. End of story."

Oscar started gesticulating wildly. "But he's been a member for *twenty years*!"

I wheeled angrily on him. "So, what you're basically telling me is this guy's been sucking cock in my sauna for the past *twenty years*? Well that's just *great*! That makes me feel a *hell* of a lot better! Now get the *fuck* out of my office!"

Despite Oscar's feelings on the subject, such indiscretions were a real problem – especially when it affected our numbers. A young Russian guy once walked into my office and announced he wanted to join, no tour or anything. He just handed me his credit card and ID and told me to sign him up. He left to go use the sauna while I prepped his contract.

As he walked away I remained motionless. My assistant stared at me. "Aren't you going to put him in the computer?"

I shook my head. "Nope, cause he's not joining."

"What do you mean? He just told you to sign him up!"

I stared sadly at the Amex in my hand and envisioned my juicy commission flying away on little plastic wings. "He's going downstairs to use the sauna – *our* sauna. You know what's going to be waiting for him. So trust me, he's *not* joining."

We sat there for barely five minutes before the kid came bursting back through my door. "Tell me you didn't charge my credit card yet!"

"No, I didn't," I said reassuringly. I handed him back his ID and Amex.

"I, uh . . . I have to think about it!" he stammered, still huffing and puffing. I nodded. "I understand completely."

As we watched, he made good his escape, looking back over his shoulder the entire time.

I can only imagine what awaited him as he walked naked in there.

Nothing like a twenty-one-gun salute.

OMG, YOU DID <u>NOT</u> JUST SHOW ME THAT!

Gay men aren't the only ones who enjoy "airing out their differences" to other guys. One day, a sales colleague decided to have some fun at my expense. His name was "Bob," and we'd worked together for some time (maybe that's why he got so comfortable).

I was sitting in my fish bowl of an office, with its glass walls overlooking the gym floor. To my left was a line of cardio machines facing downstairs. They were deliberately arranged like that to give our members something to look at while they sweated.

I noticed Bob working out directly below me, and he gestured to catch my eye. Once he had my attention, he gave a quick glance around, and then yanked the front of his sweatpants down.

It took me a second to realize Bob had gone commando, and that I was staring down at his fifty-year-old penis. I can still picture that awful, unkempt hedge of gray pubic hair. Recoiling, I gave him a look of pure annoyance before turning away.

Irritated by Bob's practical joke, I sat there scheming. I waited for him to come upstairs and then cornered him in his office.

"We've got a problem," I said. "Actually, let me change that. *You've* got a problem."

"Oh yeah," he sneered. "And what's that?"

"The next time you decide to whip it out on someone, I suggest you look around first. Someone saw you."

"There was nobody up there, I checked," he stated.

I cocked an eyebrow. "Oh really? Did you notice the girl kneeling down between the two Stairmasters, going through her gym bag? Because she sure as hell noticed *you*, buddy!"

He paled. "Are you serious?"

"Hell, yeah. She saw *everything* . . ." I smirked. "Not that there was much to see . . . She left here hysterical, crying her eyes out. Her husband called fifteen minutes ago – said he wants your head. He's calling corporate to get you fired, but not before he comes down here and punches your lights out."

"Holy shit! What are we gonna do?"

"*We*?" I shook my head. "This has nothing to do with me. *You* made this mess. Now *you* deal with it." I checked my watch. "The guy should be here within the hour."

I left Bob sitting there, nervously chewing his nails and checking the time. It was great. For the next two hours I kept an eye on him, chuckling as he jumped each time a member came in or the phone rang.

Finally, I let him off the hook. After I told him the truth he exhaled as if an elephant had been sitting on his chest, then smiled and shook his head. "Okay, you *got* me, man! You *got* me!"

I bet he thought twice after that before letting it all hang out.

At least, I *hope* so.

SURVIVAL TIP #17

Most people, regardless of sexual orientation, don't relish walking into a sauna or shower and finding two people getting it on.

I don't.

If you're offended by such things, or don't enjoy being propositioned by members of the same sex, you might want to inquire about the commonality of such occurrences in any gym you're considering joining. Don't be embarrassed to ask your sales rep.

If he or she hems and haws, you might want to check things out for yourself. Go down to the locker room, sans any staff members, and stick your head in the sauna. You might see something you don't like, but it's better to know than not know. And at least you'll be dressed at the time.

If you're already a member, your solutions are somewhat limited. If it's a one-time incident, reporting it to the club manager may resolve the issue. But if it's an ongoing problem, short of filing a complaint with the Department of Health, reporting it won't make much of a difference. In that case, your choices are limited to either avoiding those facilities or canceling and joining another gym.

You may have noticed I haven't listing grinning and bearing it as an option. That's because, in my humble opinion, most people don't appreciate going into their club's sauna wearing a welder's mask.

THE BIGGER THEY ARE . . .

Most people who work in health clubs usually end up getting fired. It's a fact of life. Sometimes they deserve it; sometimes they don't. I've seen many people get canned for doing unimaginable things. But most of those who departed did so simply because someone didn't like them and orchestrated their "demise."

It doesn't take much. A jilted receptionist with an axe to grind can easily concoct fictitious sexual harassment charges against someone (companies *dread* harassment-based lawsuits), resulting in their immediate termination. Often, the victim is let go without an investigation or any corroborating evidence.

Backstabbing is a major contributor to the incredibly high turnaround rate in gyms. Admittedly, this behavior is common in any workplace, but in health clubs it's infinitely worse. If you work in a gym, there's always someone who doesn't like you. You could be the nicest guy in the world, but the guy in the next office may secretly hate you just because you dated a girl he wanted.

You could also be the hardest-working, most punctual manager ever – someone who puts in unpaid overtime every day. Your assistant (who smiles in your face like she's your best friend) is waiting for you to do something slightly wrong so she can rat you out.

I've seen it dozens of times.

Despite over a decade with Caveat Sports, Area Manager Danny fell victim to exactly this type of thing, as did the manager of one of his clubs. It came to light that someone at his mid-town location had used a stolen checkbook to buy a slew of paid-in-full memberships. Eventually, the scam was revealed, and the company ended up with a lot of egg on their faces. They also had to refund over ten thousand dollars to the aggrieved party.

Regional Director Jack Daniels quickly seized upon this opportunity. I'd overheard him abusing Danny prior to this, and knowing how much he obviously hated him, what came next was no surprise.

A sales rep from another of his clubs had recently been arrested for being behind a counterfeiting ring that was making copies of members' credit cards. This didn't seem to matter as much to Jack; the manager of *that* club wasn't let go. But in his eyes, Danny was the one ultimately responsible for the check snafu.

Poor Danny . . . his fate was a foregone conclusion.

I'm not going to lie and say I shed a tear over my Area Manager's sudden termination – I didn't. But I did end up missing the guy. As bad as he was, we at least had a grudging respect for one another. There was a mutual understanding of sorts; at least I knew where I stood and what to expect with Danny. It was the gym version of détente, if you will.

And, as I was about to discover, the devil you *don't* know is often far worse than the devil you *do* . . .

UNTO THE BREACH

A week after Danny was terminated, I came into work to discover that Johnson, the Area Manager who ran the club in Brooklyn back when I was a trainer, was now my immediate supervisor.

I had a feeling this would not be a good thing. As I've said before, although I'd never worked for Johnson directly, I'd seen him in sadistic action a few times, and was hardly a fan. Our previous interactions hadn't ended on a cordial note, either. On top of that, I was having "political problems" on the facility front: my rigid enforcement of company policy when it came to throwing out sex offenders was making me unpopular with some of my clients and even a few staff members.

Still, I tried focusing on the positive. When Johnson showed up, I kept things professional and concentrated on running my club to the best of my abilities. Things went okay for the first month or two, but inevitably the numbers dropped. Johnson scheduled a team meeting with me and my crew to come up with a solution.

Now, unlike most managers, I was team-oriented. Caveat Sports managers have full control over who gets what (info calls, walk-in traffic, guests, etc.). Not surprisingly, most of them act like pride lions and take everything, starving their staff. That never sat right with me. I had an "everyone's gotta eat" philosophy, and spread traffic evenly. It made me popular, but more importantly it kept my team motivated.

The first thing Johnson did during our meeting was to generate fear by reading us the riot act about our numbers. We had to do something about it – *or else*. His "solution" was for my people to put in extra time and also come in on their days off – all without being paid (no such thing as overtime).

I could see my team was very much afraid of Johnson, and he reveled in using this to his advantage. He studied everyone's faces, and then stood up. "So, everybody is going to come in and work on both of their days off, as well as putting in an extra 3-4 hours each day. Anyone have a problem with that?"

Everyone stared at the floor.

Johnson turned to me. "Max, did you want to add anything?"

Looking back, I don't know why he asked me that. Maybe he was trying to make me feel like he wasn't usurping my authority, or maybe he saw my look of disapproval and figured he'd call my bluff.

I shook my head. "Actually, I'm not having my team work all those hours."

"Excuse me?"

"You heard me, Johnson. They work plenty hard already. They're employees, not slaves; they have lives. I *have* to work sixty hours a week, and that's fine. But I'm not making them do it, too."

Career-wise, it was suicide. Nobody ever stood up to Johnson, and with good reason. I could see he was absolutely livid. But I could also see the stunned sideways glances my team gave one another. And they all wanted to cheer.

"So, how do you plan on having your club hit?" he countered.

I shrugged. "We'll work harder and be more proactive. Maybe do some external prospecting. I'm sure we'll pull it off."

Johnson glared daggers at me. I could tell he was one of those people who enjoyed using his "power" to bully and abuse others. Why? Maybe he was compensating for some other "shortcoming." But whatever the reasons, he hated my guts now for having defied him. And I knew he'd be gunning for me from that point forward.

THIS MEANS WAR

Predictably, it didn't take long for Johnson to start his campaign of revenge. A manager of another Caveat Sports soon warned me that his own Area Manager had been asking questions about me. At first, he thought it was job performance-related, and sang my praises. That's when he found out Johnson was spreading malicious rumors about me, which included all sorts of nonsense. Like me being a member of a neo-fascist terrorist organization. Or maybe even being a *Republican*.

Considering that my girlfriend at the time was a prim and proper, church-going Asian girl, and my best friend was a womanizing Pakistani who smoked like a chimney, drank like a fish, and thought he was Elvis Presley on top of it; we all had a pretty good laugh on the subject.

Unfortunately, Jack Daniels was forced to listen to Johnson's incessant Max-bashing until he had to do something about it. I was called into the corporate office for a sit-down. While waiting outside, I heard Jack yelling at Johnson, "This is *your* baby, Johnson. I have no problem with the guy. So if *you* want him gone, *you* fire him. But it's on *your* head. And if he *is* what you say he is, I'd be a little *nervous* if I was you!"

Truthfully, I don't think Jack believed Johnson's poison any more than anyone else did. He was just tired of hearing it and wanted the problem to disappear.

Johnson brought me into an office and put "Alanis Blunderbuss," the company's head of Human Resources, on speakerphone. Alanis told me that my sales numbers were unsatisfactory, and that the company no longer felt I was capable of handling one of their clubs. They'd decided to demote me to a regular sales position.

Although I could tell immediately that the "meeting" I'd been summoned to was really a lynching, and that the Director of HR was in on it, I decided to stand my ground and fight. I pointed out that my numbers were better than any other manager's in the city (which they were), including gross, cash, and cancels. Then I asked her if any of the other managers were being similarly disciplined. She declined to answer, hung up, and left the rest in Johnson's lap.

When Johnson realized it was only he and I, alone together, and that all bets were off, he just sat there, sheet-white and stammering. I've never seen someone so scared. His mouth was so dry he could barely talk. When I reiterated my position, refuting the "reasons" Alanis had just listed for demoting me, all he could manage was, "But M-Max, no one wants t-to work with y-you."

I looked him dead in the eye. "No, *Johnson*, you mean *you* don't want me working for you. *My* people *love* me." I stood up and glared contemptuously at him. "I'll have to think about whether or not I'm accepting this so-called demotion. We'll talk in a few days."

I spoke to my attorney and gained some invaluable insight in regard to my situation. As a result, I was well prepared for Ms. Blunderbuss's call a few days later. She stated she understood I'd decided to accept their demotion. I told her only if I could have a sales position back at my original club (which was three blocks from my apartment).

She replied smugly, "Oh *no*, you're not going back to your old club. We're going to send you to whichever location *we* choose."

I shot back, "In that case, I'm not accepting the demotion."

Alanis was momentarily surprised, then replied, "So, you're quitting then?"

"*No*. You're going to have to *fire* me."

"Oh, we're not going to do *that*," she said with a haughtiness you could actually feel. "We're just going to put in your file that you *quit* so you can't collect unemployment!"

"Take your best shot," I said, and then hung up.

Unbeknownst to Alanis, I recorded our entire conversation. And I *still* have that tape to this day.

Sure enough, she kept her word. I got a call from the Unemployment Office – she'd informed them that I wasn't fired, but that I'd quit. I then told the agent what actually transpired (He was suitably stunned when he heard the tape).

A few days later, I got my first check.

Editor's Note: Karma has an amusing way of leveling the playing field. Although I'm not sure what became of Alanis, once I reported her blatantly unethical behavior to the New York Department of Labor, I found out her two cohorts had met with unpleasant fates.

I heard through the grapevine that, shortly after my termination, a group of women filed a class-action sexual harassment suit against Caveat Sports. Both Johnson and Jack Daniels were named as defendants. What happened to them warrants no further explanation.

I always wondered, though, if Alanis was still lurking around at that point. If so, I'd be very curious to discover what Johnson and Jack found in their employee folders when they tried collecting unemployment benefits . . .

INHUMAN RESOURCES

Based on the outright favoritism I've both witnessed and received over the years, I think "Inhuman Resources" is a far more appropriate term. Although people who work in "HR" are supposed to counsel employees, enforce rules, and assist in training and development, more often than not their primary purpose is to act as corporate headsmen (i.e. firing people while denying them unemployment benefits).

Many of them even relish the pain and anguish they inflict on others, actually gleeful in the "execution" of their duties.

I can't blame the companies that hire them; they're looking to make profits, avoid lawsuits, and cut corners wherever they can. I *will* hold them accountable, however, for the obvious partiality HR staff use when choosing their victims. Their wrath is often based on the "buddy system": upper management comes to them when they want to get rid of someone.

There was an incident at Empirical Sports where my manager Bates got carried away with one of his front desk girls. Let's call her "Bertha." Bertha was a BBW who weighed in at about 250 lbs. One day, I was standing on the member's side of our front desk, with her seated behind it. Bates walked behind the desk, his eyes focused on Bertha's considerable rear end. Without warning, he hauled back and gave her a slap across the top half of her ass that sounded like a gunshot.

I knew it hurt, because the girl yelped like a frightened Chihuahua. But since I was there, she decided to play it off. She turned coyly to Bates and said, "Oh *yeah* . . . do it again."

Bates replied (again, *direct* quote): "Oh yeah? How about if you get down on your knees and suck my fucking dick, bitch!"

For the record, this was all meant in fun, and wasn't serious in any way. Such things happen when people get overly comfortable with one another. Unfortunately, Bates had made a few enemies for himself. After a scheming employee whispered in her ear, Bertha decided she was offended and filed a complaint a few days later.

However, Bates was under the protection of the Area Manager, Peter. Peter had hired Bates – and he didn't want his protégé getting any bad press. When our HR Director called Bertha to discuss the incident, he told her, "We're not concerned about what happened. This type of thing happens at your club all the time; don't take it so seriously."

Bertha was stunned. "Oh yeah? Well, if this happened to your wife, I think you'd take it a lot more seriously."

"But it *didn't* happen to my wife, now *did* it?" came the reply.

Despite HR's cavalier attitude, Bertha kept pushing the issue.

A few weeks later, Peter came into my office and plopped down in one of my chairs. He started asking me how sales were and things like that. After a few minutes of his "foreplay" I cut him off. "Look, why don't you get to the point?"

"What do you mean?" he asked.

"What I mean is, you never talk to me and you never come into my office. You don't like me, and with all due respect, I don't like you. You're here because you've got something on your mind. So why don't you get to it?"

"Fair enough," Peter said. He studied me through hooded eyes. "Are you aware of any 'occurrences' that might have gone on between our manager and a member of your staff – a female, to be specific?"

"Is this the ass slapping incident?" I asked.

"I don't know," he remarked. "Why don't you tell me?"

I recounted what took place to the best of my knowledge and, being friendly with both parties, tried to be impartial. I could tell right away, though, where Peter's loyalties lay. He tried to play it down, suggesting it was one of those "go team" or "good job" ass taps, like you see in sports.

When that didn't wash, he reasoned that Bertha was sitting down at the time; thus, it was impossible for her to be struck on the rear end. Bates, he proposed, must have "grazed" her lower back instead.

I gaped at him in disbelief. "Are you kidding me? This is *Bertha* we're talking about. Have you seen that ass? It's huge? It goes all the way up to *here*. Her seat looks like a stool-shaped wedgie, for crying out loud!"

After a few more minutes of Peter's scheming and spinning things, I decided to stick it to him.

"Of course, the ass slap isn't your biggest problem," I announced. "It's what Bates said next."

"And what was that?"

I hesitated. "Umm . . . I don't know if I want to say it."

"I insist."

"You want it word for word?"

"Yes."

So I told him, and then watched in amusement as his head lolled back hard against the glass window of my office. He rubbed his eyes and groaned. Finally, he shook his head, thanked me for my time, and left.

Nothing was done about Bates, even with me as an eyewitness. I don't know what Peter actually reported to HR, but he must have done a pretty good job of whitewashing the whole thing, because I never heard another peep about it.

It's good being Switzerland.

THE POT AND THE KETTLE

Despite my years in the business, once in a while even I got caught off guard by things people said and did. And I don't just mean low-ranking employees, or even managers. I've seen some of the big bosses spout offensive, horrifying things – in front of witnesses, no less.

And they all got away with it.

Why? Because they were valuable.

One day, I attended one of Empirical Sports' mandatory monthly meetings. All the bigwigs were there, strutting around with their chests puffed out, bragging about how well the company's current sales promotion was doing.

Naturally, I was bored to death. Falling asleep could get a guy fired, so I kept getting up to go to the men's room. It made me wonder how many times I could slip out like that before people suspected me of having amoebic dysentery.

Suddenly, an Area Manager named "Rush" got up on stage and launched into a male cheerleader routine – yelling and screaming, trying to reanimate the corpses in front of him. He announced that the sponsors of our in-house children's program would soon be touring our clubs. Then, in front of 300 people, including his peers and bosses, he said, "Remember, it's a children's program, so they're gonna have some kids with them. So guys, keep your zippers up!"

Rush's comment hung overhead like a dark cloud; everyone wondered if they actually heard him correctly. I don't know what he had for breakfast that day – maybe some "porn flakes" with a picture of Jerry Sandusky on the box, but he offended everyone.

Was Rush fired, suspended, written up, or disciplined in any way after he insinuated we were all pedophiles?

Nope. He was a cash cow, and they needed him. Frankly, the only way he'd have gotten in trouble would have been if someone stepped forward to file formal charges against him (which would never have happened – it would be job suicide). Barring that, he probably could have spanked the monkey in front of everyone and gotten away with it.

Now *that* would be a Rush . . .

SURVIVAL TIP #18

If you work in the health club industry, you should know that a "write-up" is the standard procedure for termination so that the employee is unable to collect unemployment benefits. This is absolutely not a joke. Most of the big fitness chains have mandatory classes for managers that teach them how to successfully fire someone, while depriving them of their livelihood. They give these classes names like "Career Development." Sounds harmless enough, doesn't it?

One technique they teach is how to get rid of an employee without cause. If they have no legitimate reason to fire someone they demote them (hurting them psychologically and financially) and then transfer them to the most inaccessible location they can come up with. They'll send you to Oshkosh, as long as there's a club there. They figure, if it takes you three hours to get to work each day, eventually you'll quit on your own.

When I was a manager I was required to attend these classes. I thought the whole thing was kind of sick. There I was, taking lessons from Human Resources on how to fire someone, just so we could save the company a few dollars. Doesn't unemployment insurance come out of everyone's paycheck each week, anyway?

Ironically, most of the people in my class were eventually fired in the exact same manner, and almost always because someone higher up didn't like them. The bizarre part was, even though they were taught all about it, they never saw it coming. I guess they figured: "Oh that will never happen to me."

Guess again.

So remember: if you're working in a health club and someone throws a write-up your way, you've got two choices. Either figure out a way to fight back, or start looking for a new job. Because if you sit back and do nothing, before you know it, you're going to need one.

CHAPTER 14:

POST-TRAUMATIC STRESS

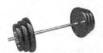

Although I'm hardly the kind to sit still, it took me four months to physically and mentally recover from my years at Caveat Sports. Between the pressure to produce, the mental abuse, and the chronic lack of sleep, working there was enough to give someone PSD. For the first few weeks I felt like I was waking up from a coma. I slept a solid twelve hours a day, just to keep my head screwed on straight.

Once I started feeling like a human being again, I extended my feelers toward my associates who still worked in the industry. My primary purpose was networking, but it seemed like every person I visited started complaining about their more problematic members. Gym managers love to gossip about all the unsavory things that go on in their clubs, even more so if the person they're talking to doesn't work for their company.

And that's when the juiciest secrets get spilled . . .

NOTHING BUT CLASS

I was in the city, visiting "Stanley," the Membership Overseer for U.S. Amazing Fitness. As we enjoyed an iced tea, while discussing sales, women, and the weather, he told me about "Belle," a young lady they just lost who had been working behind their front desk.

Belle was attractive and professional, their most trusted employee. She had the keys to open and close up – and a reputation for punctuality and reliability. The club owners eventually decided – based on her many years of loyal service – to entrust her with their bookkeeping.

Belle learned the ropes surprisingly fast; she was soon proficient enough that they allowed her to handle things on her own. Unfortunately, she had a hidden defect the owners were unaware of: she liked money. And, when given the opportunity to handle gobs of cash, she just couldn't resist putting some of it in her pocket.

Fortunately for Stanley and the owners, Belle was a neophyte when it came to embezzling. She failed to cover her tracks, and they quickly caught on to her shenanigans. Stanley admitted he was stunned when he discovered what had happened. It was impossible that his most reliable employee would turn on him like that – not after everything he'd done for her. He decided to wait until Belle came to work the next day before confronting her with the evidence.

Stanley's state of denial quickly seceded from his union. Someone tipped Belle off about the lynch mob awaiting her. Not only did she not show up for work, her phone number was disconnected. The following day, the owners went to her place with the police. Everything in her apartment had disappeared – along with the thousands of dollars of the club's cash (a severance package).

I can relate to Stanley's feeling; I had a similar occurrence at Dinar Fitness. There was a sales guy there named "Money" who was a master of embezzlement. Over a period of three months, he magically made $12,000 in cash vanish. I say "magically" because, unlike Belle, Money was experienced. He left no evidence whatsoever, and he was such an amiable, well-liked guy that no one was willing to believe he was responsible. It took six months for his crimes to catch up with him.

As certain investment banks in this country have "successfully" demonstrated, excessive greed causes many a downfall. Dissatisfied with merely ripping off his employers, Money lifted his manager's ATM card out of her wallet (after surreptitiously memorizing her bank code while she made a withdrawal). Over the next three days he systematically emptied her account of over $6,000.00.

When the manager discovered her checking account had been liquidated, she went berserk. She contacted her bank branch and ordered an immediate investigation. When they sent her the film, to her complete astonishment there was her "good friend" Money's smiling face. You could even tell from the photos that it wasn't his first dance. He'd worn shades and a hood, and kept his head turned far away from the camera. Unfortunately for him, he didn't realize there was a second one pointed right at him.

The gym owners wasted no time. After the police gave him a well-deserved smack-down (during which he also confessed to stealing the previous twelve grand), Money was given a choice: either cough up the cash or spend the next five years in prison. He called everyone he knew, even yours truly, asking to borrow it. In the end, his parents grudgingly coughed it up and Money took his vaudeville act elsewhere.

NOW *THAT'S* GRATITUDE FOR YOU

When you work in a health club, you interact with a wide assortment of clientele. Rich and poor, thick or thin – I've seen them all. I've dealt with drug dealers and degenerates, whackos and wiseguys, doctors and dentists, harlots and homeless (I once signed up a vagrant by convincing him it would give him a chance to stay warm, not to mention the use of our showers and toilets), and everyone in between.

Along the way, I've done favors for hundreds of people. When you're forced to manipulate peoples' emotions all day long, it feels nice to do a good deed every once in a while. Especially if your actions have a direct impact on someone's life – possibly even saving it. Clients always remember things like that, and if you run into them in a restaurant or on the street, they're always happy to say hello.

Well, *almost* always . . .

A few months after I'd "quit" Caveat Sports, I stopped by my old club to visit "Apollo," its current manager. Apollo was quite the character – a ladies' man whose charm and good looks were only exceeded by his substantial ego. He was a born salesman, a crafty manager, and a compulsive liar.

When I got to the club, I observed Apollo struggling with a very irate member – an elderly gentleman who kept waving a handful of papers in his face. From what I could glean, there was a problem with his contract. Apparently his renewal rate was much higher than he expected. As I looked harder, I realized I recognized the guy; it was the same old man I'd saved a year or two earlier from what I called "death by sauna."

I remember heading toward the pool area, when a member emerged from the sauna. As the door closed behind him, I saw the older gentleman lying motionless on his side. Even from a distance I could tell something wasn't right. I went in to check on him – and found him burning up and unresponsive. I had no idea how long he'd been there – or how many people (both members and staff) had come and gone without giving him a second glance – but he was completely dehydrated and suffering from heatstroke. I hoisted his naked, eighty-year-old body up and carried him outside (trying to ignore his wrinkled genitalia resting on my forearm). After calling 911, I administered a few cool compresses and waited for the EMTs.

Luckily, the oldster lived. He never came back to say "thank you," but that was fine. I was sure he'd be happy to see me now.

Boy was I in for a surprise.

As I headed toward him with a big smile on my face, the old man spotted me and screamed at the top of his lungs, "You! You're Max! You screwed me!"

I stopped in my tracks. I had no idea *what* the guy was talking about. A fierce argument ensued; he snarled and snapped at me in front of the gawking staff and patrons. After a few minutes, I grew tired of his abuse and my temper got the better of me. I called him an ungrateful relic with raisins for nuts and that I regretted not leaving him in the sauna. He could have turned into a mummy, which would've been great because we could have propped him up as a warning to other members on how *not* to use the sauna.

Apollo wisely ushered me outside. After failing to put a damper on my self-righteous indignation, he decided to derail my steam train of a temper by coming clean. It turned out *he* had enrolled the old man a few years prior, but the geezer couldn't remember the last time he'd used the men's room.

To save his own skin, Apollo told him his contract was *my* doing – that *I* was the one who lied about the rates.

At first I was pissed. But then I waved the whole thing off. I couldn't stay angry at him for lying like that. It must have seemed like a safe bet; I no longer worked there, and once blame had been assigned, there was no absolutely way to hold me accountable.

Unless I just so happened to walk through the door at that very moment . . .

YOU'RE *WELCOME*

I'm reminded of another, less-than-grateful client I had back at U.S. Amazing Fitness, I was standing outside my club, enjoying the crisp night air and taking a well-deserved breather from the phones and treadmills. It was fairly late, and with my club being situated on a quiet, one-way street on the Lower East Side, the hustle and bustle of the day was pretty much over.

All of a sudden, "Brook," a prim and proper blonde I'd just enrolled, came out of the club and struck up a conversation with me. I was tired and not feeling particularly congenial at the time, so she did most the talking. My contribution consisted of an occasional nod or grunt, just to be polite.

Eventually, Brook realized I wasn't in the mood to chat and went to cross the street.

The fact I wasn't paying attention to her saved her life.

I was standing by the curb, with Brook to my right. A delivery van had pulled up by the hydrant, thirty feet to my right, and was sitting there with its engine running. I don't if some Jedi-like sixth sense warned me, but I *knew* what was coming. As Brook stepped off the curb, the van's back-up lights came on and the driver reversed at high speed. I lunged forward, grabbing her jacket's rear collar and giving it a powerful yank.

I was just in time.

The van's side panels whooshed past, inches from Brook's nose, and it stopped right where she was standing. It was a scary moment. The girl would have ended up a mangled mess, pinned underneath the vehicle, midway between the axles.

The driver paused for a second, then threw it into gear and sped powerfully forward. I leaned in close and whispered, "*That* wouldn't have been good."

As the van burned rubber and made good its escape, I released my grip. Brook's weight shifted forward, and she staggered into the street. Without a word, she walked stiffly away. I noticed her gait had a bizarre stagger to it, like her joints didn't work right or something. I don't know why; maybe it was from all the adrenaline. Or maybe she'd experienced a different kind of "accident."

The next time I saw Brook, she didn't even mention her near-death experience – let alone thank me. Instead, she went to my Area Supervisor and complained about my "attitude." I literally saved her life, and that's how she repaid me.

It just goes to show, "no good deed goes unpunished."

GUESS WHAT WE FOUND IN YOUR LOCKER?

When I became manager of the Caveat Sports in Manhattan, the commute had been a serious annoyance. My old club was only three blocks from my apartment, and I enjoyed training there more.

That being the case, I decided to keep my old locker there. It was nice – and big enough for you to hang a business suit in. To make sure my belongings were secure, I had the maintenance guy drill out the clasp, enabling me to use a padlock more suited to a tractor trailer than a gym locker.

Apollo, my successor at my old club, knew all about my locker. When we were colleagues and I was still an employee, he had no problem with it. But once I'd left the company (under less than auspicious terms), he decided to take it back.

I got a phone call from Apollo, complaining that his guys had tried and failed to cut my lock. The hasp's steel was so hard and thick that their bolt cutters could hardly get around it. Of course, the trainers he assigned were undeterred by this; they tried cutting it two at a time, one of them hanging from the big bolt cutter's handles.

Once the locker clasp was twisted beyond recognition, they lost their composure and physically beat my padlock with the cutters. After ten minutes of this chaos, they finally succeeded in removing it – but it was the clasp that gave out, not the lock.

The funny thing is, if Apollo had just asked, I'd have happily come by and removed my belongings. Instead, they ended up annihilating a steel locker door, leaving them with a pricey repair bill.

I was told to come down and get my stuff. When I got there, my bag – and everything they'd been able to jam into it – was waiting in an office. Sitting on top of it in plain view were several dozen condoms, all shiny and ready for action, like a bandolier of sexual bullets.

Apollo's current Assistant Manager pointed out that when they wrenched my locker open, a huge shower of condoms fell out. She thought it was quite the spectacle – and apparently expected me to be terribly embarrassed. She didn't realize she was dealing with someone who could sing Lou Bega's *Mambo Number 5* without substituting any names. Why would I *care* that they knew I used to bang members in the club after closing? I didn't even *work* there anymore. Not to mention everyone else was (and is) still doing it.

I smirked at her, grabbed my bag and my rubbers, and said, "Cool. I can really *use* these . . . Thanks!"

Then I left, leaving her and her friends with their jaws hanging open.

ABSOLUTELY PRICELESS: THE CUSHINETTE

A few days later, I swung by another Caveat Sports club to meet a colleague for lunch. While I was waiting at the desk, I ran into an aerobics instructor I'd worked with in the past. Unlike my other peers, my interaction with instructors was fairly limited. I never bothered taking any classes, and for the most part they simply came in, taught and left.

This particular instructor, however, stood out. Her name was "Toni," and she was what I call a burnt-out disco queen – a Brooklyn chick who had her heyday back around *Saturday Night Fever* and hasn't changed an iota since.

Not her clothes, hair, makeup – nothing. It was like she climbed out of a time capsule.

I overheard Toni bragging to some members about a date she'd gone out on the night before. Before I could escape, she grabbed me by the arm and asked if I'd tried out the fancy restaurant she was talking about. I was in a rush, but she was very persistent. When I admitted I hadn't been there, she proceeded to rave about the guy that took her there and how wonderful the food was.

Toni gave a wistful look toward the heavens, took a deep breath and touched her hand to her heart. "Oh God . . . the *cushine* was delicious!"

I blinked confusedly, and then shook my head. "It's *cuisine*, you *moron*!"

Toni stood there, wallowing in confusion as I walked away. I paused for a moment, wondering if maybe I'd been wrong. I mean sure, in my eyes, the woman had the brains of a goldfish, but knowing the neighborhood she came from – as well as the general lack of morality that pervaded that club – maybe she was right.

Maybe the guy *was* delicious.

ON MY COMMAND, UNLEASH HELL!

After hearing about the lawsuit that cost both Johnson and Jack Daniels their jobs, I decided to pop in on Apollo to toast their demise. Unfortunately, he'd already left for the day; so with nothing else to do, I decided to use the club's restroom before leaving.

When nature calls, you have no choice but to answer the phone. And my line was *really* ringing, if you catch my drift.

The nearest restroom was inside the gym's woefully undersized nursery. I checked my watch; luckily, daycare hours were over, so I seized the opportunity. The "bathroom" they had for the kids was as proportionately small as the rest of it. At my size, I could barely squeeze in.

I squirmed inside and discovered my stomach cramps were a prelude to the worst case of diarrhea I've ever had. This was an eruption like Mount Vesuvius; anything within range of that toxic cloud would've been killed in seconds.

After a good ten minutes of wreaking havoc, I managed (after some twisting and writhing) to stand up and flush. To my horror, the toilet was clogged (before I got there, I assume), and the water began to rise, its vile contents eagerly seeking freedom. I'm sure most of you have experienced this terror at least once in your life; you extend your hands and ineffectually scream, "Stop!" as if it would make any difference.

Panic set in. As there was no toilet lid to slam shut, I did the manliest thing I could think of: I fled, shutting the door behind me.

Through the closed door I could hear the sound of water spilling over the edge of the toilet and cascading down onto the tiled floor, plopping noises that suggested unspeakable horrors.

Completely terrified at this point, I crept out of the nursery. Fortunately, no one was around. Rather than pass the receptionist again and risk her connecting me with the crime scene, I snuck through the nearby aerobics studio, then took a set of stairs that allowed me to pop out from an emergency side exit. The alarms on those doors never functioned when I worked there, and thankfully still didn't.

Like a burglar fleeing a botched robbery, I made my way onto the street and vanished into the crowd. For the next three blocks I fought down the urge to glance back over my shoulder – fearing that at any moment the Caveat Sports Police would come charging after me, the front desk girl screaming, "That's him. He's the one! Get him!"

Fortunately, I made a "clean" getaway.

Six months later, I was hanging out with Apollo. When I recounted my tale to him, he was shocked. He told me about "Leonid," who worked there – a huge, oversized bodybuilder. Leonid had a history of flatulence and a reputation for causing people in the locker room to flee for their lives when he did his business (steroids and high-protein diets will do that to you). The manager and his staff automatically blamed Leonid for my misdeed and gave the poor guy so much abuse over the next few weeks he finally threw up his hands and quit.

In retrospect, I gained some perverse pleasure from destroying my old club's bathroom like that. It was a fitting bit of revenge, if you will. I felt like I'd done to Caveat Sports what I've seen them do to clients all these years.

CHARACTER SPOTLIGHT: KONG LIVES!

Eventually, I started looking for work in earnest. One of the first places I interviewed with was a chain in the city called "Crash Fitness."

I took the train uptown, toured the place, and met with the manager. I wasn't impressed with the location. The layout was confusing – a lot of small rooms that made the place seem more like a maze – and the air quality was poor. What really stood out, however, was the manager, himself.

Let's call him "Kong." He was 6'5" and weighed about 350 lbs, with most of it stored around his midsection. Not exactly a paragon of health and fitness, if you know what I mean. On top of that, Kong wore a pair of cut-off sweatpants and a matching sleeveless sweatshirt, which not only showed off the pale, fur-coated slabs of fat that made up his arms, but also his bloated, hairy stomach – which peeked out at me from beneath its straining fabric.

As Kong interviewed me, he went on about adjusted gross and numbers, and bragged about what a selling machine he and his team were. He showed me a huge binder that contained what he called "dead leads," i.e., the tour cards of people who never joined, but whose info was still on file. When things got slow, his sales reps made follow-up calls to these people, even if it was a year later.

I guess in Kong's primeval world, if you don't take "no" for an answer, it'll pay off, eventually.

As our interview continued, I noticed a young sales rep in the next office finishing up with a well-dressed couple. They didn't join, but they seemed pleased and shook his hand enthusiastically before leaving. Kong rose to his full height and asked the rep why they didn't sign. The guy nervously said, "They want to think about it, they'll decide by tomorrow."

Kong's face turned ugly, and he snatched up the dead leads binder. "Nice job, loser," he snarled, and then threw it at the poor guy. As the binder struck him hard in the chest, Kong added, "Why don't you make yourself useful and go make some calls?" The rep, obviously frightened, sat down and did just that.

This spectacle was enough for me. I'd never work for any company that'd hire an oversized buffoon like that in the first place. And I *certainly* wouldn't take his abuse. I'd have left that place in handcuffs, probably with one of his ears dangling from my teeth. Of course, wouldn't you know it; he tried offering me a job.

I deliberately told him, "I'll think about it."

The next day, Kong called and tried to push me into accepting his offer. His VP had apparently heard of me (at the time I had quite a reputation), and wanted me hired ASAP. I told Kong I was flattered, but I'd given the matter some thought and the answer was "no." He became very flustered and started rambling that he "didn't have time to waste if I wasn't serious about coming to work for them," and that he was "behind the 8-ball" because he still had "'X' number of dollars of sales to do that day."

I told Kong he was lucky I *wasn't* working there, because if he'd thrown that binder at me I'd have shoved it up his hairy ass (again, that's a direct quote). He choked on his anger and surprise, grunted like a wounded cow, and then hung up on me.

There's never a squadron of biplanes around when you need one.

SURVIVAL TIP #19

After that last experience, let me emphasize again: If you're considering joining a health club, keep in mind that whatever tour card you're requested to fill out will ask for a lot of personal information. This is not for the company to track its advertising, as you'll be told, but so your sales rep can follow-up with you if you don't join. You may want to substitute the number for your dry cleaner or local Chinese restaurant, because if you don't sign up, you'll get calls until the day you die.

I was never one of those guys who keep haunting potential clients – after an attempt or two I got the message – but I've seen reps call the same lead every day for two years. Can you imagine being afraid to answer your own phone, deleting voice mail after obnoxious voice mail for two years?

Take my advice. If you don't have a disposable number to use when you start shopping for a health club, be prepared to change the one you have. Because if you don't, there's a good chance your name (and number) will end up in the "dead leads" file.

And stay there.

CHAPTER 15:

BACK INTO THE FRAY

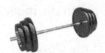

After the requisite six months of unemployment, I found what would end up being my favorite job in fitness. I ended up as the Membership Director of a small, privately owned chain in the city known as "U. S. Amazing Fitness."

My prior years at Caveat Sports had really taken their toll – not just physically, but spiritually. I'd seen so many negative aspects of the health club industry that I had become jaded. Luckily, my new employers were different; they were a non-corporate outfit and their gyms were all family-owned. From what I could see during my initial tour, the floor staff were all very happy with their jobs – a good sign.

More importantly to me, the owners were appreciative and supportive of their sales team. Maybe they knew what I'd been through and wanted to make me positive and productive; maybe they were just smarter than my old bosses. Either way they gave me free reign to run my own show, and wisely sat back while I did it. I was also blessed with being able to work regular hours. Instead of putting in sixty or more stressful hours per week, I was only required to work forty. And it was a *relaxed* forty, at that. Best of all, though, was the money: salary-wise, I was making *twice* what I did at my old job.

No stress, a third less hours, and twice the money . . . I can't think of a better way to renew someone's dwindling faith in their career.

THE PINNACLE

In addition to all the other perks at U.S. Amazing Fitness, there was also an undeniable female factor. As a consummate ladies man, being surrounded by beautiful women could only brighten up my day. And the women who lived and worked around my club were absolutely amazing.

The Lower East Side attracted visiting hotties from all over the world, most of them on three-month travel visas. I met girls from Japan, Finland, Estonia, Australia, France, South Africa . . . you name it. I couldn't be happier. Because of all this positive "motivation," I also got back into a formal workout routine. Proper training and dieting was the name of the game, and within a few months I'd lost any and all extraneous body fat. I was in tip-top shape, looking and feeling great. Plus, with the money I was making, I could afford to buy some decent clothes.

Looking back, I was truly in my glory.

My improved self-image also had a tremendous impact on my selling prowess. Besides my appearance, my positive emotional state was apparent to every client I worked with. It was hard for someone to have reservations about my club when I literally came out dancing to greet them, smiling ear to ear.

Meeting a cheerful employee is like seeing a happy child – you know right away that whoever's in charge is doing a damned good job.

Week after week and month after month, I rocked the house. I broke every sales record the company had, and set some that stand to this day. The owners thought I was the greatest thing since sliced bread. They used to joke about cloning me so I could work all their other clubs at the same time. I can't tell you how many times I heard, "Oh Max, you're so wonderful. You're such fun to work with, and you make us all *so* much money. We just *love* you!"

ABSOLUTELY PRICELESS: THE BIG SHOT

Besides working for better people, my new clientele were a step up, too. They were friendlier and more relaxed, as well as easier to talk to. And not *once* did I witness someone shaving their testicles in the sink next to me.

This was undoubtedly due to the neighborhood, along with the fact that the club itself was cleaner, cooler, and better kept than any I'd ever worked – a benefit of having no bureaucracy and owners who took a hands-on approach to maintenance.

Not all of my clients were nice, however.

One day, a well-dressed, middle-aged couple came in. I could tell right away, based on the $5,000 suit he was wearing, that the guy was some sort of corporate big shot – a CEO, or some such animal – obviously strong-willed and intelligent, and certainly not someone to play mind games with. I decided to take the sensible approach and be straightforward and direct.

I introduced myself and offered to show them the club. As we started onto the gym floor I turned to the husband and asked, "So, what kind of equipment are you looking for?"

It was a fair question, and I hoped, once he saw we had everything he needed, he'd consider joining. He turned to me with a nasty look and said, "Can you do us a favor?"

"Sure . . ." I replied. ". . . If I can."

"Can you *not* talk to us?"

My eyes narrowed. "Excuse me?"

"You heard what I said," he remarked. "You see, we don't want to hear your sales spiel or any of your bullshit. We just want to see the gym and then leave." He looked me in the eye. "Do you have a *problem* with that?"

I felt my temper rise and weighed the ramifications of what I was about to say.

"Actually, yes, I *do*," I said with a cool smile.

"Oh yeah?" he replied.

"Yeah . . ." I gestured around the club at my members. "You see, this is a family-owned business. And these are all very nice people. Frankly, I don't think you're going to fit in here."

"What? What's that supposed to—?"

"It means you need to go find another gym," I interjected as I pointed a thumb back toward the lobby. "I trust you can find your way out?"

His eyes popped and his face turned beet red. "How . . . how *dare* you!" he sputtered.

"Oh, I *dare* alright," I said through my teeth. I noticed the look of astonishment on his wife's face as her jaw took a break on her chest. She'd obviously never seen anyone stand up to her rude and abusive husband before. "Have a nice day."

He stomped off toward the lobby, then wheeled back around and shook his fist at me. "You haven't heard the last of this!"

"Oh, I hope I *have*!" I fired back.

I always wondered if that guy worked for Lehman Brothers . . .

SURVIVAL TIP #20

This one applies to both members and employees. Clients like the last one are the stereotypical troublemakers who often cost health club employees their jobs. They're rude, nasty, and consider themselves beyond entitled. Someone like that will frequently complain to management or even the corporate office; they will try and use their power and position to extract some measure of satisfaction, if not outright revenge.

I guarantee this guy contacted my club's owners to complain about me. I expected it. In fact, I called them myself as soon as he stormed out the door, just to cut him off at the pass and let them know what actually transpired. Fortunately, I had a great relationship with my employers. "Don't worry, Max. We have complete faith in you. Whatever happened, we're sure you did the right thing, and we back you 100%."

Keep in mind, that type of response is the exception, not the rule. If I'd gotten that type of feedback from my Area Manager at Caveat Sports, I'd have had a heart attack and died on the spot.

If you're forced to deal with a blowhard like that, best to keep your cool and be as professional as possible. And try to make sure there are witnesses around who can back up whatever is said – otherwise, Lord knows what they'll make up.

THE MISER

Nobody is perfect, and "Rodney," the owner of U.S. Amazing Fitness, turned out as imperfect as anyone. Rodney had several flaws, but his biggest was that he was the fitness world's greatest miser. I didn't know it at first; the guy was always generous with me. But then again, that was in his best interests. I was bringing him at least a million dollars of business a year, which undoubtedly had an impact.

I did know, however, his wife was stingy. I took a cab with her once, and had to ask the driver to wait a full ten minutes while I unloaded a bunch of presentation materials. I promised him a good tip, and Rodney's wife said she'd take care of it.

Later, I found out she gave the poor guy exact change.

One day, Rodney came into my office and showed me a check. This was back in 2006, and the check was dated for 2005. When I pointed this out he grinned and said, "Yeah, this cheap bastard I signed up around this time last year gave it to me and it bounced. So I changed the five to a six . . . see here? I'm thinking he's probably forgotten about it by now, so I'm gonna redeposit it and see if it clears."

As I cocked an eyebrow, Rodney smiled and clapped me on the shoulder. "See, Max. Now you know what a greedy bastard I am."

And he was *not* kidding.

LA SERPENTINA

Rodney had one additional flaw. He had too much faith in my immediate supervisor, aka his District Manager, "Britney."

I'd known for some time that Britney was the only worm hungrily gnawing its way through my otherwise perfect apple. She was an aggressive woman who, although nice on the surface, had a very dark interior. Several times, I'd watched her confront trainers suspected of doing sessions under the table. Each time – despite a complete lack of evidence and their vehement denials – she fired them on the spot. And she was completely vicious about it – yelling, screaming, and threatening. She threw them out of the club immediately, withholding their final paycheck as well. These people had been with the company for years, productively doing their jobs for satisfied clients, but when she got the idea into her head that they were skimming, she cut them off like they were nothing.

Britney was also a highly sexual creature. She shared stories of her dalliances with me many times, including her obsession with being thrown around by big black men ("Max, there's *nothing* like it!"). She'd slept with many members of her staff, including trainers and housekeepers. One time, she even started making eyes at me. She was a little surprised by the Max-shaped hole I left in her door.

I'd never slept with a "superior" (and still haven't). And, considering her bony frame, nasty temper, and wanton promiscuity, I wasn't attracted to

Britney in the least. The bottom line is, of all the bosses I've ever had, she was the last one I'd have gotten it on with.

And that includes the guys.

One day, Britney called all of us into her office for an impromptu announcement: "Empirical Sports Clubs has just purchased this gym. They'll be here in thirty minutes – you're all out of a job."

My day took a sudden, downward spiral after that.

In my mind, I saw my whole world enveloped by a fiery nuclear blast.

As I sat there, reeling from this unexpected development, Britney threw me a life preserver. Although they'd sold most of the U.S. Amazing Fitness clubs to Empirical Sports (mine included), Rodney and his wife had kept one for themselves. And they wanted me to stay on doing sales there. Britney said, "We're all family and we love you so much that we want you with us."

Caught off guard as I was, I agreed to stay and didn't ask any questions. I probably should have. Especially this one: "Which club was Rodney keeping and why didn't Empirical Sports want it?"

If I knew the answer, I might well have reconsidered their generous offer.

WHERE THE BOYS ARE

To my surprise, it turned out that, according to Britney, Empirical Sports passed on purchasing Rodney's sole remaining U.S. Amazing Fitness club because they were "homophobic." The club was in Chelsea – and had a reputation as a Mecca of gayness. There were well over 5,000 members – 95% male, and 99% gay. And this included the staff.

I was stunned. Unlike my old location at Caveat Sports, where the members kept their preternatural sexual activities on the down-low (at least outside of the steam room and sauna), at this club, the members couldn't care less what people saw. To them, it was their private Roman bath house. They would make out at the front desk like it was required, and hooked up wherever and whenever they got the opportunity. One housekeeper complained to me that every time he checked on the sauna, guys were getting it on left and right – with others masturbating while watching. He lamented that they were always "in mid-stream" whenever he opened the door, and that he had to constantly clean up their ejaculate-laden towels.

I suppose it didn't help that half the guys were escorts.

It was quite a bit of culture chock for me to adapt to this radically new environment. Since nothing was being done by either the owners or management to curb the full-scale orgies (they said they'd lose 25% of their business if they did), I avoided the steam room and sauna like the plague.

Sales-wise I was doing fine – partially because word had spread about the tall, hunky "straight guy" working there. I guess it was quite the scandal; members were insatiably curious about me. The resultant attention was definitely good for business. Guys brought me friends to join just so they had an opportunity to sit in my office and talk. Maybe they thought they'd be able to "turn" me or something . . .

Despite being surrounded by a host of oversexed gay men, I was never hit on. Not even in semi-private situations like selling in my office. That's usually the case. For some reason, gay men don't tend to come on to me. I don't know why; maybe I'm just not "hot enough," or I give off the wrong vibe. Or maybe I'm just so oblivious to their flirtations that they fly right over my head.

However, one day, while I was getting changed in the locker room, my luck finally ran out. I'd just finished a particularly pathetic workout and was really annoyed about it. I'd recently blown out my shoulder and was unable to train with weights, at least upper body-wise. As a result, I'd put on a few pounds, and my jeans were getting tight. As I wrestled my way into them, I uttered a grunt of disgust.

As I did, I heard a soft voice with a very pronounced lisp ask. "What's wrong?"

I looked to my right. Seated on a nearby bench was a, well . . . *fairy*, for want of a better word. I swear if I looked closely, I could see Tinkerbelle-like wings. I knew the guy – at least on a first name basis. "Tinker" had developed a habit of coming into my office to buy personal training packages, so naturally I was nice to him. I assumed it was because he went through a lot of sessions.

Turns out I was mistaken.

"What was that?" I asked.

"I asked what's wrong," Tinker said. "You sound upset."

"Upset? Hell, yeah. I'm a fat slob, and I can't fit into my pants."

"Oh, I think you're *gorgeous*."

Reality took a header out the nearest window, and I stared at the lockers in front of me, thinking, *"Did he just say that?"*

"You are *so* much hotter than all the guys walking around here who think they're God's gift," he continued. Then, as I stared in disbelief, he clasped his hands together like a little schoolgirl praying, and added, "I've waited two *weeks* to tell you that!"

Little cartoon hearts were hovering over his head.

I had no idea what to do. It was totally unknown territory for me, and I didn't know whether to be angry, embarrassed, or flattered. It wasn't like the guy reached over and grabbed my ass, and I felt bad for him, since he was definitely barking up the wrong tree.

Finally, my hard drive crashed, and I gave him a blank stare.

"Nice *weather* we're having . . ." I said. Then I walked out, leaving him sitting there.

The guy was so "miffed" he never spoke to me again.

Years later, when that club finally changed owners, its sauna and steam room were closed down permanently by the Board of Health. The new management had no choice. They were unable to control the rampant sexuality of their members and couldn't afford to have that type of inappropriate behavior going on for the whole world to see. I remember seeing the story in the paper. The headlines read: "Sauna closing leaves gays steamed."

It was a catchy title.

PORN TO BE ALIVE

Amusingly, the most perverted client I had to deal with during my last few weeks at U.S. Amazing Fitness wasn't some horny gay guy cruising for some action. It was a relatively straight, former adult-entertainment star who went by the name of "Randy Rugburn."

Randy was just a wee bit on the outgoing side. He told everyone about all porno movies he made, the thousands of women he had intercourse with, the venereal diseases he caught, the drugs he used, and even the times he overdosed. He had a maniacal sense of humor, would say anything to anyone, and came up with the filthiest subject matter imaginable. He enjoyed making a spectacle out of himself, and loved that some people tried to avoid him for it.

One day, I spotted Randy talking to one of my front desk girls. For no apparent reason, he asked her for a cup of water. I ordered her not to do it, but she didn't listen. As soon as she handed Randy the cup, he dumped it on our freshly waxed lobby floor. I cursed and reached for the overhead mike to call housekeeping. Before I got the chance, the culprit stripped off his t-shirt and lay down in the puddle he'd created.

As I stared, Randy used the skin of his back and the water to form a seal on the smooth tile. He flexed his back muscles while lifting his hips off the floor, making the loudest and most offensive flatulation noises I've ever heard. As he did this, he screamed things like, "Oh God, dude, take it out! Take it out!" and "Oh man, sorry, that chili was good!"

I couldn't believe I had a grown man lying on the floor, behaving in this manner, while other members were checking in less than ten feet away. Meanwhile, my receptionist lay on the floor in a fetal position, cackling hysterically with tears running down her face.

Another bad habit Randy had was talking dirty to people while he dry-humped them. He'd do it to just about anyone who allowed it, male or female. A lot of guys there got a kick out of this, and the rest were too shocked or embarrassed to fend him off. I, on the other hand, was used to his antics – so when he tried it on me, I sent him flying.

Unfortunately for Randy, he was slow to get the point.

A few days after the floor incident, he popped into my office. I rolled my eyes and got up to leave. As I did, he crept up behind me, then latched onto my hip and started humping my leg. I tried to shove him off, but I had no leverage – he was locked on like some sex-starved, 250 lb. Saint Bernard.

At the time, I used to carry a small folding knife in my pocket. It was a nasty little thing – tiny – but so sharp you could shave the hairs off your arm. Best thing about it, though, it was a legal auto-opener – like carrying a switchblade, but without the obligatory jail time.

As Randy continued to rape my thigh, I suddenly remembered my knife. I made a final, ineffectual attempt to free myself before exasperation took over. My temper flared and I gave a quick glance around. Then, in one smooth motion I drew it free and slammed him into the nearest wall. The instant he hit the drywall, my blade was at his throat.

"You should learn to keep your crotch to yourself," I hissed.

Randy's eyes bulged in fear, and I think he pissed himself. "Y-you're fucking crazy, man! Y-you could lose your job for this! Y-you could g-go to jail!"

In a split second the knife was closed and back in my pocket. "Go to jail for *what*?" I asked. I gave him a warning look. "*I* didn't see anything. Did *you*?"

Suffice to say, the guy kept his penis away from me after that.

A dog may be man's best friend, but in these days of super-strict handgun laws, an easily accessible blade has *got* to be a close second . . .

Editor's Note: Do NOT follow my example. Carrying a weapon of any kind at your job, even a "legal" one, is cause for immediate termination. Although I might have convinced the cops I was being sexually assaulted, I could just have easily been arrested for assault and battery.

ET TU BRUTA?

After two weeks of working at my blatantly gay club, the place was wearing on me. Feeling uncomfortable while changing or taking a shower was not something I could get used to. Nor could I adapt to needing galoshes in order to enter the steam room or sauna, or the shock of walking in on two or more guys doing their interpretation of Michael Jackson's "Beat It."

The final straw, however, came in the form of Britney, my supervisor. Before Rodney sold his gyms, her job was to oversee his clubs while I ran my location's sales. Since Britney's salary was predicated on my success – she received no commissions herself – she was supportive, even generous at times. Once there was only one club, however, things changed. Britney had made an arrangement with Rodney wherein she not only got commissions from sales she did, but also a cut of the club's net profits.

She began taking steps to increase her cash flow. She started by cutting her sales team's salaries in half, followed by our commissions. Then she started stealing our clients and signing them up herself. Finally, her true nature began asserting itself during team meetings, and she repeatedly tried to debase and abuse me and other employees.

That was it for me. The next day, I started going on job interviews during my lunch break, and within a week I found a fantastic sales position at a chain called Dinar Fitness. I was through dealing with all the responsibilities and pressures of being a manager – no more of that, thank you very much. I could make just as much money doing sales, without having to cope with all the bullshit. That following Monday, I called in sick and tried out my new gig. And the next day, I told Britney I wasn't coming back. With no notice, mind you.

Editor's Note: Knowing that my employers would never give me my last paycheck, I played it smart. The week before, I asked the owner to pay me my year's vacation in advance. I told him I wasn't going to physically go, but I didn't want to lose the money.

That evened things out between us, more or less.

SURVIVAL TIP #21

As someone who experienced this first hand, take it from me: if someone cuts your salary or demotes you the way I was, legally you're allowed to up and leave. And, you should be able to collect unemployment benefits with no problem. Based on what I was told by a rep from the Department of Labor, the substantial loss in earnings significantly affects your lifestyle and your ability to support yourself. Hence, you're allowed to quit and collect while looking for a better job. A lot of gyms don't want people to know this; if they did, it would put a serious crimp in their ploys to force people out.

CHAPTER 16:

SEX, LIES, AND DUCT TAPE

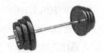

took the job at Dinar Fitness with the hope of finding a new home. I wanted a place with good people, like I had when I began working at U.S Health and Fitness, but with more room for growth. I started at one of the Dinars in the city, but soon transferred to one of their Brooklyn locations. My newfound club was impressive. Although it didn't offer a pool or Jacuzzi, it was huge, with lots of perks and amenities. There was even a parking lot.

I immediately put my sales abilities to work. It took me a week to learn the ropes. During my first full month, I took 3rd place in the entire company. It was 1st place from that point forward. My bosses loved me because I was doing what they loved: making them money.

I WANT YOUR SEX!

My new job was a nearly perfect setup. It was close to home and it paid well. My one "complaint" (if you'd call it that) about working there was the overt sexuality of the place. It was a heterosexual version of the U.S. Amazing Fitness location in Chelsea. Everyone was obsessed with two things: their appearance, and whom they could sleep with next.

Almost all my clients had a membership at a local tanning salon. Every guy was on steroids (more on that later), and every woman wore next to nothing. The girls had more makeup on than clothes. I'd never seen a woman train in high heels before I came there. And breast implants? They were the norm. Once, I saw a woman who'd just had hers done. She was on the gym floor, and as I watched, she pulled up her shirt and showed her brand new DDs to all the guys, so she could get their opinions (which they were only too happy to give).

The place was *totally* out of control.

The complete opposite of this overt exhibitionism was a gay guy who frequented the men's locker room. They called him "the Camcorder Guy." He'd stroll around the locker room carrying his gym bag. Inside it, he'd concealed a camcorder, with nothing showing except the lens, discretely peeking out from one end. He'd walk around, talking to guys and making small talk, while filming their asses and genitals.

One day, Camcorder Guy got busted. The members he'd victimized didn't take kindly to being part of his home movie collection. They beat the shit out of him, smashed his camcorder, threw his wallet and keys down the sewer, and then tossed him out the back of the building, buck naked.

Mind you, this was February. Amazingly, the guy didn't press charges.

Maybe he didn't want his wife finding out.

The staff at Dinar Fitness was almost as bad. A receptionist working there by the name of "Nymph," became obsessed with the idea I was well-endowed.

Editor's Note: Note, I said idea . . .

One day, as I was changing in the nursery (while it was closed, for sure), Nymph tried bursting in on me. She was very sneaky about it. She had the key and waited outside until she figured she had a good chance of catching me with my pants down. Then, she slid the key into the lock and flung the door open in one, smooth motion. Her cry of, "Omigod, Max, I'm so sorry!" sounded a little hollow. Especially when I noticed the way she was "covering" her eyes. She had her fingers spread wide, for what she hoped would be an unobstructed view of my manhood.

Fortunately, I'm a quick-change artist and was already dressed. I was a little annoyed, though. And it wasn't because she weighed over two hundred pounds. Her live-in boyfriend was a good friend of mine, and he wasn't thrilled when I told him what she'd been up to.

Another time, I discovered one of my fellow sales reps was banging one of our personal trainers. That may not sound so bad, but the fact that they were doing it in the club during prime hours was a bit of a no-no. Whenever the mood struck him, "Lance" would grab "Lancet," and after a half-hearted struggle on her part, drag her bodily into the nearest closet or "pump room."

Apparently, this had been going on for months.

I witnessed their bizarre courtship one day. As I watched, Lance grabbed his victim and hauled her toward a nearby storage room. Lancet saw I was watching and must have been embarrassed, because her struggles were more fierce than normal. I heard Lance grumble in frustration, "Why don't you just be a lady and let me beat the shit out of you?" The next thing I knew they were in the cleaning supply room, right next to the gym floor.

Unable to pass up the opportunity, I crept to the closet door. I could hear the sounds of stuff being moved around, along with the rustle of clothing being removed. I waited another minute or two, then grabbed the doorknob and shook it like an earthquake. I had to bite my tongue to keep from laughing when I heard their muffled cries of alarm; Lancet's cheeks were definitely rosier than normal when she crept out of there a minute later.

Even the managers at Dinar Fitness were big-time perverts. One of them once gave me a great demo on how he ran the club. At the time, "Goon" had a crush on the current Fitness Manager – a short-haired Russian girl with a "J-Lo-style" rump that was hard to ignore.

Goon took "Rumpzilla" out for some "external prospecting." It turned into a more *internal* kind, because they ended up back at his place, snorting down a whole bottle of vodka in the middle of the day. A few hours later, he dropped Rumpzilla back at the club and asked me to come out to the lot. I had to hold my breath to avoid a contact high from all the booze on his breath, while listening to his tale of sexual conquest. He told me to run the club for him for the rest of the day before driving home to pass out.

When I went inside, Rumpzilla was nowhere to be found. I assumed she'd also snuck out and went home. Later, when I used my key to enter her office, I found out she'd crept into her closet to sleep it off. When she heard the door open, she came staggering out, fearful she was going to get in trouble. When she realized it was "only me" she teetered to and fro, babbling on and on about how drunk she was. Then, she gave me this coy look and asked me to lock the door to her office so we could check out the inside of her "closet."

I passed; I do have *some* decorum, after all. Not to mention that I would never touch anything someone else just had their "hands" on, most especially my oversexed boss.

SURVIVAL TIP #22

Just a refresher course about the perils of dating health club employees: remember, most of them are promiscuous, regardless of whether they're in a relationship or not. I had a receptionist at Empirical Sports who lived with her long-term boyfriend. He paid her bills and their rent, he put food on the table – but she was still dating the world behind his back.

I noticed a string of guys hanging out by the front desk whenever she was on shift. When I asked her about these men, she admitted she was dating them – all of them. After I got over my initial shock and asked her exactly how many guys she was seeing, she told me, "Oh God . . . I don't even know how many guys I'm dating; there's that many."

That's a direct quote. So remember fellows, like the man says: "Don't be a fool, wrap your tool."

BREAST WISHES

Highly sexual members and staff can be bad enough. But when you throw in the subject of "real versus fake," with a club's nursery as the battlefield, you're asking for trouble.

There was a very busty young lady working out at Dinar Fitness known as "Candy." I call her that because that's what she seemed to consider herself.

As I mentioned, Candy was especially curvaceous above the waist. As such, the staff and members regularly debated whether her "girls" were implants.

One day, Goon called me into the nursery (again, it was closed at the time). He was with Candy, who was proudly posing with her hands on her hips and a gleaming smile on her face. Goon explained the rumors that Candy's breasts were fakes and brought it to her attention. Candy was outraged. She proclaimed to us, in no uncertain terms, that her breasts were 100% homegrown and natural.

When Goon stated he wasn't fully convinced, Candy volunteered to show us. Before I could utter a, "Whoa, let's shut the door!" she'd hiked up her shirt, unhitched her Brooklyn Bridge of a bra, and exposed her massive mammaries for both of us to admire. She even allowed Goon to squeeze them, just to make sure there were no doubts in his mind. I passed on the opportunity. Not as much from a gentlemanly impulse, mind you, but because I figured the girl was nuts. I didn't want some BS sexual harassment charge being thrown at me, should she fall in a bad mood.

LIGHTS OUT!

I once had an interesting experience with a client whom I'll forever refer to as the "Light Fixture Lady," or "Fixture," for short. Fixture was a young single mom who came into my office with her sleeping infant in tow. The little boy, maybe six months old, was nestled in a removable car seat. Two chairs for clients were positioned directly in front of my desk.

Fixture sat the baby (in the car seat) in the chair to her right, and then plopped herself down in the remaining chair. As we started to speak, a metal light housing suddenly fell out of the ceiling over her head. It impacted hard on the arm of the infant's chair (narrowly missing his tiny head), before landing with a thump.

I was horrified and jumped to my feet to make sure the baby was okay. Fortunately, he was untouched and remained blissfully asleep. I examined the light housing, which was aluminum, circular, and fairly heavy. Moreover, its sharp edges had cut a groove into the hard plastic of the chair's armrest.

As I examined the housing, I told Fixture, "Thank God this didn't hit your baby." Then I made the mistake of blurting out, "Because if it had, you'd have owned this gym."

I regretted my words instantly. A wild look came over her, and as crazy as it sounds, I think she was actually considering whacking her poor baby over the head right then. Her eyes jogged back and forth from the baby to my hands, and back again. I could see the wheels spinning in her head. It was a dangerous moment. I think the only thing that stopped her was my alert expression and my grip on the offending piece of metal. She must have realized I'd never go along with it. And that I'd have physically stopped her.

Amazingly, when I went to my manager to express my concerns, he paid Fixture's behavior no mind. Instead, he took the aluminum housing, got up on my desk, and reinserted it. Then, to make sure it was "safe," he slipped in a paperclip so it wouldn't fall again. *A paperclip.*

I told my co-workers about the incident. They pointed out that many of the lights in our offices were hanging loose in their sockets; some seemed poised to come plummeting down. It was a running joke from that point forward: whenever entering one another's offices they'd push the door open as hard as possible, in the hopes of one of them getting bonked.

CHARACTER SPOTLIGHT: MISTRESS MAYHEM

In addition to irrational parents, you also need to watch out for your club's resident dominatrix.

Officially, dominatrices are women who take the aggressive, "dominant" role in fetish-style bondage and/or sadomasochism. Based on my "experience," they tend to frequent gyms – not just to stay in shape, but also to acquire submissive men interested in their particular talents. Just about every club I ever worked had at least one dominatrix lurking around. Some were on the DL (down low), whereas others were quite overt and even bragged to me about their "clients," and how much they charged per "session."

Possibly the most brazen "dom" I ever encountered was at Dinar Fitness. We referred to her as "Mistress Mayhem," or "M&M" for short. I'd heard many stories about M&M, even from my General Manager. Once, she hid in the ladies locker room until after the club was closed. When he came down to do a sweep of the place there she was, wearing nothing but a towel around her waist and eagerly offering to tickle his prostate.

He told me he said "no."

M&M had a crush on one of my regulars, a pretty boy known as "Maybe."

One day, Maybe and a bunch of his friends were hanging out by the front desk. Since Maybe considered himself far too good looking for M&M, he ignored her groping advances and kept yakking away with his buddies.

Out of nowhere, the girl uttered an inhuman grunt and pounced on him. In front of a dozen stunned witnesses, she picked him bodily up off the floor and tossed him toward the front door. Then, despite his struggles, she hauled him into the tiny men's room adjacent to my reception area.

Word spread about what was going on, and within seconds a dozen people piled into the narrow hallway outside the men's room, climbing over each other to listen in on what was "going down." We heard a fierce struggle, along with some whining on Maybe's part, followed by M&M's distinctive voice saying, "Oh c'mon, baby. You know you want me to take charge . . ."

After that things got pretty quiet and we couldn't hear anything. A minute later, some killjoy hauled back and kicked the bathroom door as hard as he could.

Nothing happened. There was no lock, so the only thing we could figure was M&M had her victim pinned tightly against the door. A few minutes later, the sink started running, and everyone bolted for the front desk, trying to look as innocent as possible.

Mistress Mayhem strutted out of the men's room wearing an ear-to-ear smile. She made a big show of wiping her mouth with the back of one hand,

and then walked proudly down to the gym floor. A minute later, Maybe emerged to find a score of us staring at him. He turned red and ran out the door like his feet were on fire.

We changed his name to "Definitely" after that . . .

THOU SHALT NOT COMMIT . . .

Dating fellow gym members can be fun and exciting. The main reason why people join health clubs in the first place is to meet fit, well-endowed members of the opposite sex.

Unfortunately, a lot of people looking for action aren't always honest and upstanding. They'll lie like a rug to get what they want. And it doesn't matter whether they're male or female. An aerobics instructor at one of my clubs once had to transfer to a different location after she found out a cop she'd been sleeping with was married with children.

She found out when the guy's infuriated wife showed up and informed her in front of a bunch of people – and not too quietly.

Adultery is commonplace, if not the norm. I don't know if it's a sign of the times or the general lack of morality in this country, but it's an everyday thing. I once witnessed a confrontation involving a man and two women at my front desk. It turned out the guy had been sleeping with both of them (one was his wife). The wife had initiating the fight, but not because of her husband's faithlessness. She had been sleeping with the *other* woman's husband, and was angry because *that* wife was interfering with her extramarital "relationship." She wasn't concerned about her *own* marriage (if you could call it that). She just wanted to keep having sex with the other girl's husband and was furious she wouldn't let her.

Most amazing, *her* husband (the one standing there) seemed perfectly fine with all of this. I, on the other hand, was left with no choice but to send them packing.

Why?

Because, from a sales perspective, few things compare with the potential family-of-four you've got waiting patiently by your front desk, overhearing, "So, your wife fucked my husband, and you're *okay* with that?" from one of your members.

Not exactly an ideal setup for a positive selling experience . . .

The most extreme, adultery-fueled brawl I ever witnessed, however, took place at an Empirical Sports club. The instigator was a fit European woman named "Sophia." Sophia had an accomplished reputation for cheating on her husband. Sophia's opponent was her former best friend, "Lauren." The two women had stopped talking a few weeks prior. Lauren told me she'd grown tired of Sophia ringing her doorbell at 2 a.m., asking to drop her off so her husband would see the two of them coming home together.

Things came to a head when Sophia accosted Lauren in the gym. Her current "boyfriend" wasn't returning her calls, apparently because he liked Lauren. The two of them got into a terrible argument on the gym floor; Lauren denied the allegations and berated Sophia, calling her a whore.

Lauren tried to walk away, but Sophia followed her into the women's locker room. The confrontation escalated as they were changing, and the two started the world's greatest catfight. They were rolling around on the floor – punching, kicking, and clawing like two naked mountain lions. Seconds later, four more women wearing nothing but towels came rushing out of the steam room to break up the melee.

I got involved when two girls in towels came running up to me, screaming, "Help! You have to do something! They're killing each other and we can't stop them!"

As I rushed into the women's locker room I was treated to the sight of a half-dozen scratched-up, hot, naked women in a dog-pile on the floor, screaming, struggling, and cursing at one another in languages I couldn't begin to understand. I had to figure out what was safe to grab onto as I prized them all apart.

Let me tell you, I've had far worse days.

SURVIVAL TIP #23

If you're dating a fellow gym rat and not looking for adulterous complications, it pays to do your research. Start off by asking. Surprisingly, a lot of married men and women will tell prospective lovers up front about their situation. Although they might claim otherwise ("If only I'd met you first, darling . . ."), this is done primarily to make it more convenient for them to cheat. It's a lot easier to sustain an adulterous relationship if your lover is supportive of your situation. Then you only have to lie once.

If you suspect the person you're dating/considering dating is married and they deny it, a simple background check should tell you everything you need to know. You can do it online in a few minutes. Better to invest a few dollars and a little time than to find out the hard way via an enraged spouse...

SHOCK AND AWE

You'll occasionally come across people in health clubs whom you'd be much better off avoiding.

Few people really scare me, but "Lilith" from Dinar Fitness was definitely one of them. It's not that she was ugly; in fact, she was tall and attractive. But she also could say the filthiest, most disgusting things imaginable. She could make a New York City cab driver blush – and got off doing it.

When I was giving tours I avoided Lilith like Chernobyl.

I learned to do this the hard way.

One day, I was taking a young college guy around. He was very enthusiastic about joining, and our tour was pretty much a formality. I spotted Lilith standing by our circuit training machines, along with a half dozen other clients. She was buxom, and he was a young buck, so I decided to stop for a quick "hello." It certainly couldn't hurt. As I introduced my client, Lilith gave him a half-hearted smile and then turned her sights on me.

"So, you know Mark and I got engaged," she announced.

"Congratulations," I said. "I'm happy for you."

"*I'm* not," Lilith remarked. "I don't wanna fucking marry him!"

"Then why are you?" I asked, suddenly conscious of my client standing right beside me.

"Because none of you assholes would ask me out!"

Embarrassed, I tried mollifying her with a flirtatious grin. "Oh, c'mon, baby . . . you know I'd have gone out with you in a *minute!*"

It was a bald-faced lie, of course. There was no way I'd go anywhere with a short tempered, foul-mouthed hellion like that, but she didn't need to know it.

Unfortunately, my tactic backfired.

"Oh no, you *wouldn't*," Lilith stated. She moved so close to me I could feel the heat radiating off her body; I swallowed nervously as she stared me down from six inches away. "You wouldn't *fuck* me the way I want you to. You just want to leave a hot load in my *mouth!*"

I froze in place, my eyes the size of teacups. I didn't know what to do. All around me I felt the scrutiny of the nearby people, most of whom I didn't even know. I cast a sideways glance at my client, then stared fearfully back at Lilith.

"Um . . . have a nice day?"

It was all I could come up with before retreating for the safety of a near-by stairwell. Fortunately, my fears of losing a sale proved to be unfounded. My client was actually entertained – if not outright aroused – by Lilith's antics, and even more motivated to join.

Thank God for testosterone.

AND THE ABUSE JUST *KEEPS* ON COMING

As entertaining as Lilith was, there are plenty of members who enjoy belittling and tormenting health club employees. Some people do it out of a warped sense of humor, whereas others are just plain vicious, cruel, or frustrated with their lives.

One time I took an elderly grandmother on a tour and ran into a regular named "Mack." I'd known Mack since he was sixteen. He'd been a fan of mine since my Caveat Sports days, back when he first started lifting and looked up to me as a bodybuilding god.

Currently, however, Mack had developed an annoying habit of trying to embarrass me by making freakish comments as I showed customers around. Knowing this, I would have steered clear of him, but he caught me off guard by popping up off a bench from only forty feet away.

"Hey, Max," he shouted loud enough for half the gym to hear. "How's that rash doing? The one you went to the doctor for; did it clear up?"

Praying my potential client's hearing aid needed batteries, I retaliated. "Oh, you mean the one your *sister* gave me? Yeah dude, tell her it's cool!" (For the record, Mack's sister was very hot – and had also dated a good friend of his behind his back – so my rebuttal was spot on).

I had another member who shared my passion for fishing. Let's call him "Rags." Rags was a corporate sales rep who used to come into my office every day to talk about fishing trips and charters – and his fancy new boat. Although we never fished together, we got along great.

Or so I thought.

One day, right after I bought *my* first boat, I took a moment to tell Rags about it. Even though it wasn't as big or glamorous as his, I'd designed it myself, so I figured he'd appreciate it. Especially after all the times he'd talked my ear off on the subject. When I told him about all the modifications I'd done to it, including having the name emblazoned on its hull, he sneered at me and said, "Oh yeah, with what . . . spray paint?"

I paused and gave Rags a cool, calculating look. The kind you give someone you *thought* you knew after realizing they're a complete jerk. I didn't say a word, though. I just shook my head and walked away, leaving him standing there.

Editor's Note: In retrospect, that explained why he'd bragged to me about spending fifteen grand on a new outboard for his boat, instead of buying an engagement ring for his long-suffering girlfriend . . .

A few days later, I had my last encounter with Rags. He snuck up behind me outside the men's locker room and tried to spook me. From the sadistic grin he was wearing, he must have thought it was pretty funny. Unfortunately for him, I didn't. As he sprang out at me, I got up in his grille and informed him, "The next time you pull something like that, I'm gonna take you outside and fuck you up."

He stared at me uneasily. "Oh yeah?"

"Oh *yeah* . . ." I repeated. When Rags looked in my eyes, he knew I meant business. He got scared and walked away, and he never spoke to me again.

FOWL PLAY

Like I said, a lot of people like to give gym staff grief – not just the members. Even visitors get in on the action. One time I was forced to deal with a nasty pair of would-be guests at Empirical Sports. As I walked up to the front desk, I could hear them giving my receptionist a hard time. Apparently they didn't want to pay any guest fees, and they weren't being very nice about it.

To avoid a confrontation, I explained our policy to them in a very professional manner. One guy didn't want any trouble – he stayed quiet and kept hanging back. His friend "Mouth," on the other hand, had a real attitude and started getting belligerent.

"I'm sorry, Mouth," I said. "But that's the fee. You also have to fill out a guest sheet and leave your license."

"Forget it," he said. "I don't pay guest fees."

"Here you do. Sorry."

"Fuck that. I have a Caveat Sports Clubs membership. I don't need this place, and I don't pay guest fees!"

"Then you don't come in. Rules are rules."

"Who do you think you *are*?" Mouth shouted, trying to make a scene. "Do you know who I am? Do you?"

"No, I don't," I answered, annoyed. "Why don't you tell me?"

"I have friends at *corporate*! I don't pay guest fees! You're letting me in and I'm *not* gonna pay!"

"No, I'm not."

"I'm gonna call corporate! I'm gonna have your *job*!" Mouth screamed.

"Go ahead," I said. "Take your best shot." Then I added, "Oh, by the way, your guest fees just went up. They were $15.00 each. Now they're $25.00."

Mouth got so close I thought he was going to stick his tongue in my mouth. His rancid breath washed over me as he bellowed, "You know what you are? You're a *nobody*!"

"And you're a *wannabe*," I replied with a smirk. I was sick and tired of dealing with this guy. It was time to end things. "And now you *can't* come in."

"Oh yeah?" he glanced past me at the gym floor. 'You gonna stop me?"

I gave him an evil smile. "Oh, I don't have to do *that*. You and your girl-friend have exactly thirty seconds to leave my gym. If you don't, I'm gonna call my cop buddies and you two ladies are going to leave here with a pair of lovely silver bracelets as a parting gift. And, as a bonus, since it's Friday evening, you'll get to spend the weekend with some *very* pleasant company."

By the time I'd walked into my office and pretended to dial the phone, the two of them were in Hoboken.

SURVIVAL TIP #24

If you ever have to deal with characters like the ones I just mentioned, you need to develop either a very thick skin or an un-shakable, Buddhist-style philosophy. Otherwise, you're liable to lose your temper and do something stupid.

That doesn't just mean going G.I. Joe on someone and beat-ing them senseless (which would lead to you being arrested, fired, and sued – in that order).

By blowing your stack, you might say something regretta-ble, which is exactly what people like that want. By dropping to their level, you play into their hands. Like most corporations, in the fitness industry, the customer is always right (unless they owe money). Especially when they've got something legitimate to complain about or file a lawsuit over.

Stay strong, keep calm, and quote regulations to no end. With enough practice, you can find a way to "stick it" to most people. Best of all, you'll never have to hear about it from your boss, except perhaps for a grudging acknowledgment that you followed company procedure to the letter.

Sometimes being a good little soldier can come in handy.

CHAPTER 17:

BIG NAME, BIGGER PROBLEMS

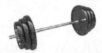

ife has a funny little way of making things come full circle. Some people call it prophecy. When my boss at Dinar Fitness announced that
Empirical Sports had just bought out our facility, I called it, "What the fuck?"

Once more, a corporate giant, bent on expansion and conquest, had
disrupted the stability of my little world. I'd finally gotten myself a high-pay-
ing job close to home, and despite all the sex maniacs roaming my club's
halls (or maybe *because* of them), I was fairly comfortable. Now, *again* these
people were screwing things up for me. No matter where I went I couldn't
seem to get away from them.

After some deliberation I decided that "if you can't beat 'em, join 'em." I
was burned out and figured that, maybe this would turn out to be a good
thing. After all, Empirical Sports was an up-and-coming leader in the fitness
industry, with at least a hundred fancy locations throughout the country.
With that kind of pedigree, how bad could they really be?

They certainly charged their customers through the nose. Maybe they'd
pay me more!

So I rolled the dice and accepted their offer to retain my current position. All I could do was hope I didn't end up with craps.

DO AS I SAY, NOT AS I DO

My new employers were basically no different than the people back at
Caveat Sports – petty, vindictive, and backstabbing. The only difference
was, perhaps, that they were more pretentious and condescending. That,

and the fact that the memberships now cost a hell of a lot more for the exact same facility.

Disregarding all that, I focused on doing my job and staying out of trouble.

Unfortunately, trouble often has a way of finding you.

My first Area Manager at Empirical Sports was a tall, seemingly pleasant woman named "Jeanette." Although she seemed nice, there was something about her that made me uncomfortable. She had a habit of making vaguely sarcastic remarks with a beatific smile, which made it impossible to tell what was truly on her mind. I've always known that a skilled assassin will smile in your face right before they stick in the knife. And Jeanette certainly struck me that way.

At Empirical Sports, all the sales staff and managers had to work the last day of the month, even if it was their day off or a weekend. The only exception to this was if the rep, club, and company had all already hit their respective quotas. In that case, should the "closeout" fall on your day off, you could stay home.

Since it was my first month, the policy was still a little hazy to me. As it so happened, the last day of the month fell on a Saturday, and I couldn't come in that day anyway. After suffering a heart attack, my father had sold his house and needed to get his belongings out ASAP. Many of these items were extremely heavy, and he needed my help.

I explained the situation to Jeanette. I was sure that, given the circumstances, she'd understand – especially since it was still three days before closeout and I had already crushed my numbers. The club had already hit and the company was about to. She gave me a hard time anyway, saying I was "ignoring company policy" and "not acting like a team player." "It's the 'principal of the thing,'" she said. I was stunned. She'd have my father drop dead from struggling with furniture if it meant she could get a bigger bonus.

When I stuck to my guns and told her that I absolutely needed the day off, she said, "Do what you have to," and smiled in my face. I soon found out why. She didn't want to risk ruining my club's sales flow for the end of the month. She wanted me motivated and upbeat for the next two days – and waited until that following Monday morning to call me at home and suspend me. She also told me that I'd receive a write-up, although I never actually got one. Maybe she was nervous about what I'd write in the comments section, or maybe she just forged my signature and stuck it in my file.

It wouldn't surprise me.

The following month sales weren't as good, and my club was faltering. Come the last day, we still needed more than twenty memberships to hit. My manager was out sick, and while getting something from her desk I discovered a hidden cache of certificates for the company's "Family & Friends" membership promotion.

I had struck gold. Technically, each staff member was only allowed to sell two of these discounted memberships, and then only to close friends and family, but desperate times call for decisive action. My coworker and I grabbed the whole stack and went on a world-class selling binge. We called people up and pitched them like it was a one-in-a-lifetime special – which, given the fact that they technically weren't entitled to it, it was. It was like shooting fish in a barrel. Between the two of us, we enrolled thirty people over the phone in less than three hours – and all but one was effectively an "illegal" membership.

Our club triumphantly hit the numbers that month, and we got big bonuses, too. Strangely enough, Jeanette, who kept daily reports on all the memberships sold at her clubs, never said a word about the mysterious influx of "family" members who joined that day. I guess "company policy" and the "principle of the thing" didn't apply when it came to the bosses. Either that or Jeanette's vision became suddenly impaired when her own ass was on the line.

HERE TODAY, GONE TOMORROW

During my years at Empirical Sports I discovered that the company had an astonishingly high turnover rate.

Regardless of their position, people came and went faster than the seasons. I barely got to know them before "*poof!*" they were gone. If you've ever been to a gym, you know exactly what I'm talking about. It seems like every time you come to exercise, you'll see a different person behind the front desk, an unfamiliar trainer on the gym floor, and a stranger sitting in the offices. Most clubs change managers more often than their members change their oil.

There are many reasons for this high turnover rate: pathetically low pay, abysmal treatment, and the piles of stress.

The salaries most fitness chains pay are substandard. Minimum wage is the norm, and many places will pay less if they can get away with it. The only way you can make decent money is in sales, which is totally cutthroat and comes with a ton of pressure. And no matter what position you hold, expect no loyalty from your employer. Everyone is expendable to the invisible suits up above, and the higher-ups treat their underlings like dirt because they know they can get away with it. If anyone objects, soon enough they'll be fired and replaced. Anyone who can't hack the abuse and quits will get replaced, too.

The origin of this mass exodus is at the very center of the apple – the companies themselves are literally rotten to the core. I'm not talking about whatever concepts or ideals they were founded on. *It's the people.* Everyone in gym management has worked their way up the same "corporate ladder," kicking and clawing their way up its slimy rungs over the mangled bodies of their colleagues. After growing callous and apathetic, they treat their staff badly – and pay them even worse – because that's how it's supposed to be. Because it's how *they* "made it," everyone else should suffer the same ordeal. When an abused boy grows up and has a child of his own, his innate tendency is to behave the same way his dad did. Subconsciously that's how he thinks things are supposed to be.

They're not.

Because the staff is so mistreated, it's next to impossible for a gym to hold on to quality people. How hard do you expect someone to work – scrubbing floors, cleaning toilets, picking up trash, and dealing with a shitty boss – for $6 an hour?

Let me tell you – it *ain't* gonna be very hard.

As soon as I became a manager, all of these problems were obvious. Unfortunately, there was nothing I could do about it. I argued for improvements that would be better for the club and the company, both long and short term, and make more money overall. My pleas fell on deaf ears. They couldn't care less that I'd put in more than a decade in the front lines, or that I'd dealt with a hundred thousand people.

I was a "grunt." What could I possibly know?

Gyms need people with morals and character – people who are dedicated to their jobs and love the industry they're in. But that would cost the owners more money, and *their* only interest is lining their pockets. Background and qualifications don't matter, as long as the bare minimum gets done.

Empirical Sports literally once hired a used car salesman who bragged about selling lemons to single moms with kids. The company didn't care; all that mattered was whether he could close. It never dawned on them that this character would lie to his customers, and even cheat his own club to get his commission. Sure, he got caught, fired, and replaced with the next charlatan – but until then he was a cash cow, which was all that mattered.

Hiring bad people is a vicious cycle, one that's almost impossible to stop.

BALL BREAKER

"Peter," one of the Area Managers at Empirical Sports, was a perfect example of the corporate culture. When I first met Peter, I wasn't sure what to expect. He was extremely well dressed, and gave off an impression of being a consummate professional. When I smiled and shook his hand, however, I found out otherwise. As he gave me "the grip," I realized that, for whatever reason, he was sizing me up.

Although we rarely had to interact, I saw him at work quite often. I learned very quickly that the guy was mean, pure and simple. One day, he noticed someone had plugged a cell phone into an outlet behind the front desk and demanded to know whose phone it was.

I could tell instantly that "Sunny," my receptionist, was familiar with Peter. Teeth clenched, she nervously admitted it was hers. Without another word, he ripped her phone and charger out of the wall and flung them at her. With a spiteful sneer on his face, he spat, "Well, you're not using *my* electricity!"

What was the problem? The juice couldn't have been more than a few pennies – Sunny was a hardworking single mom who needed her phone to work.

And how was it *his* electricity? I didn't remember seeing "Pete's Gym" on the signage outside. Regardless, that's how the guy was. He was like my old boss Johnson, back at Caveat Sports. Pete enjoyed hurting people and spreading fear. It was like he was compensating for something.

He was. And I eventually found out what.

Peter's wife was an extremely controlling woman. *She* was the one who wore the pants in the relationship, pure and simple. Since he couldn't be the "king of the castle" at home, he took his frustrations out on everyone else at work. It was his chance to be in charge. At work, *he* was the big Kahuna, and everybody below him paid a hefty price for it.

Whenever he disliked someone, he would organize a campaign to fire them, gathering documentation until he had sufficient cause to cost them their job. I clashed with him constantly, especially after he started gunning for my boss.

One day, I had a bit of fun at Peter's expense. When I showed up for work I found find him seated in my boss's office, drinking coffee and sending emails. Sunny was acting very strangely: she paced back and forth behind the desk like a caged lion hyped up on amphetamines. And she openly and hatefully glared at Peter as if she didn't know I was there.

I asked Sunny what was wrong. As soon as she opened her mouth, I knew she was high on something. I don't know what drug she'd taken, but her eyes were wild and glazed over, and her lips moved non-stop as she spoke. Something was also going on with her jaw, like she was lip-synching in a badly dubbed kung-fu movie; her teeth kept chattering for a second or two after each sentence.

She pointed at Peter. "*That* mother-fucker (*chatter-chatter*), I've got a bone to pick with him (*chatter-chatter*)." Eager for some entertainment, I encouraged her to go speak with him. She grumbled that she couldn't because she didn't have coverage.

Kind and generous soul that I was, I offered to man the desk for her.

Two seconds later, with drool dribbling down her chin, Sunny stormed into Peter's office. She flung open the door – slamming it so hard that she cracked the drywall. He jumped up with fear in his eyes. She loomed over him and bellowed, "You and I have a *serious* problem, mister."

Unfortunately, she slammed the door closed and I was forced to rely on visuals from that point forward.

QUID PRO HO

Another thing I noticed at Empirical Sports – and in the fitness industry in general – was that people would do anything to advance themselves. I was never surprised by the lows they were capable of stooping to.

Well . . . almost never.

One person there really stood out in this regard. Her name was "Widow." Widow was a General Manager for one of the clubs in my region, an attractive woman with long, dark hair and nice legs. Given my penchant for dark-haired beauties, I might have been interested in her myself, but she was already involved with "Bates," my current manager. Officially, as colleagues, their relationship was verboten, so they tried keeping it hush-hush. Unfortunately for them, Bates made the mistake of sending me into his office to read something off his computer and had inadvertently left his email open.

The banter going back and forth between them left little to the imagination.

I teased Bates mercilessly for this, not realizing he'd go crying back to Widow about it. She sent me several hilarious emails after that, which described how much she couldn't stand me and accused me of being "jealous" of their relationship.

A few months later, Bates resigned and Widow set her sights on a more ambitious target. She struck up a friendship with Peter, our Area Manager. They were hardly discreet, and juicy rumors began to spread. It didn't help when Widow was foolhardy enough to public fawn over Peter's "sexy tattoo." Of course, their intimacy didn't go over too well with Peter's wife. She showed up unannounced one day and straightened her husband out in front of half the gym.

Shortly after that, I was passing by the manager's office when "Sal" (Bates' replacement) had Widow on speakerphone. She'd just landed herself a highly sought-after job – and knowing her relationship with her boss, a lot of people wondered how she got the "position." Sal was one of them.

Widow bragged about her elevation from "lowly" management into corporate. She also boasted about how easy the gig was; she no longer had to worry about quotas and was making even better money than before.

Sal noticed me loitering outside. He gestured for me to come into his office and shut the door, but cautioned me to keep quiet. With the door closed, he continued his conversation with Widow.

"So, that's some new position you got yourself, huh?" he said.

"Yes," Widow replied. "It's amazing. I'm making even more money and have almost no responsibility. I absolutely love it."

Sal winked at me, and then flat out asked, "So . . . how many dicks did you have to suck to get it?"

"Just one," she answered without hesitation.

In my mind I could see Widow down on her knees as she "interviewed" for the job. A wave of nausea came over me, and I signaled to Sal before quietly getting up and leaving. As I walked toward my office and pondered this latest bit of information, it blew my mind that this was all it took to get a juicy promotion. I couldn't help but wonder: If I'd been born a hot babe – considering my charisma and gift of gab – would I be CEO of my company already?

Ironically, a few months after she'd "moved on up to the east side," Widow was suddenly given a final written warning and then summarily fired. I don't know the precise how or why, but I heard rumors swirling around about someone's angry wife making a big stink about things, and that the same someone had to cut their losses.

Maybe that was true. Maybe it wasn't.

Or maybe Widow's "performance" simply wasn't everything she thought it was, and they found someone better equipped to fill her position.

GOOD GOES BAD

The pressure to perform takes a mighty toll, and in my field it brings out the worst in people.

During my last few years at Empirical Sports, there was an unpleasant incident during one of our monthly closeouts. It was nearly 9 p.m. Only a few minutes were left on a high-pressure twelve-hour shift that capped a long and exhaustive month. We still needed a dozen more sales to hit, plus a few more to stave off the inevitable trial-cancels. Anyone could tell it just wasn't going to happen.

My normally laid-back boss, Antonia, was reeling from all the pressure and abuse coming down from corporate. Not wanting to accept grim reality and disappoint them, she was on my ass like a diaper.

Now, "Isabelle," was a hard-working single mom with a one-year-old daughter who looked forward to getting back in shape. I'd already spoken to her earlier in the day, however, and found out that her baby was sick. She wanted to wait a few days so she could bring her daughter with her (to make sure she'd be okay in our daycare). Her money-back guarantee would start then. I knew better than to pressure her. From a monetary perspective, it didn't matter to me whether she joined that day or in five. Her commission would still be in my next check.

Antonia, on the other hand – desperate to pull in some last-minute sales – asked me to call Isabelle again and pressure her into "not missing the sale." I pointed out that it was late in the day, and that the woman had a sick child. Antonia was insistent; despite my objections, she ordered me to make the call.

The results were disastrous. The ringing phone woke up the poor, sick baby (I heard her wailing in the background), and Isabelle was furious at our lack of consideration. So, instead of gaining a new customer – as would have happened if my instincts and common sense had prevailed – both the company and I lost one, making an enemy to boot.

Forget the money! I felt absolutely awful. The bullies up in corporate could turn even Antonia into a ruthless reptile. All that for just one lousy sale.

How greedy and grasping could they be?

I had to do some serious soul searching at that point. It made me realize the price I was paying for working there.

THE HEAD OF THE SERPENT

Shortly afterwards, something happened that forever cemented my views of both Empirical Sports and the fitness industry as a whole.

The CEO of Empirical Sports, "Matt Jones," was a fan of mine. I'd turned down repeated offers to move up in the company, but Matt knew I loved my club and my people. He also knew that I had my finger on the pulse of things, so he made it a point to drop by every six months or so to pick my brain (what was left of it).

I was always happy to see Matt; he was my last and final hope that the reasons I first started working in fitness weren't some pipedream. He believed in our product more than anyone and spread the word of the benefits of proper exercise and nutrition. I personally showed him around whenever he popped in, and gave whatever feedback I could. (To prevent him from being harassed, I told everyone he was an architect who worked for the company)

Toward the end of what would be Matt's final visit, I decided to pitch him a radical sales idea I'd been working on. I proposed a system wherein the company gave residual income from each membership sold ($1 per month per sale) to the salesperson who closed the membership. This would last as long as the client stayed a member and the rep was employed. The best part was it wouldn't cost the company a thing – all they had to do was to time it with their next dues increase and raise their dues (one time only) one extra dollar. I calculated – with the average membership lasting 2+ years – that these "residuals" would eventually cap, but they would make every sales rep work *much* harder to build up what would end up becoming, to them, a nice monthly bonus. It would also give them something to fall back on after losing commissions during vacation time.

The system would attract better, smarter, more honest, and harder working reps. It would establish more sales "anchors" at each club, increase employee retention, reduce turnover and training costs, improve customer service, and even reduce cancelations. Hell, it's amazing how hard a salesperson will work for a lousy dollar.

I was very excited about my idea and hoped Matt would see its inherent value. I wasn't looking for a promotion or raise. I just figured it would be a great way to build the business and spread fitness.

Matt looked me up and down, then said, in his inimitable Australian accent, "Well, Max, that's an interesting idea, and it's good to see you're thinking long term. But if we could squeeze an extra dollar out of these people, *we* would deserve it!"

"<u>We</u> would deserve it…"

I recoiled and then stared at Matt like he was a big, ugly spider I'd just found crawling through my kitchen. With an involuntary "Ugh!" I walked away, leaving him standing there.

Although that was the last time I saw Matt, it didn't matter. The damage was done. The guy ran one of the biggest fitness chains on the planet – one with hundreds of thousands of customers. I looked up to him because I believed that, of all the people I'd known, he actually cared about his customers.

But I was wrong. In the end, the only thing he really cared about was the same thing that everyone else did: money…yours and mine.

"Squeeze an extra dollar…"

To this day, Matt's words still echo in my head. In those two sentences he exposed the fitness industry's ultimate philosophy. Then and there, I lost the tiny bit of faith I still had in the industry. I knew, once and for all, that I was slaving away for people who pretended to promote wellness, but whose real agenda lay in milking their customers.

From that day forward, I focused on taking care of business. Not for myself, mind you, and *certainly* not for my employers. I concentrated on helping my customers to the best of my ability, even at the company's expense. And I don't regret an iota of it. If there was an angle or loophole that would save my people money, I'd find it and exploit it – even if it made me less cash. And my customers *loved* me for that; in fact, it turned out to be the secret of my success.

At the end of the day, gym owners are making a big mistake. Despite what execs like Matt Jones think, the American public isn't stupid; they're just not all as well-informed as they could be. And it is the ill-informed who fall prey to their assorted schemes.

Hopefully, this book will change some of that.

CHAPTER 18:

TERRIBILIS FACILITATE

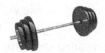

Terribilis Facilitate: Latin for, "Fearful Facility."

It's time to take a break from my anti-establishment rants and focus instead on some of the more dangerous things I've seen in health clubs. This includes gym injuries, violence inside and outside clubs, and (if your location has one) parking lot perils.

Also interspersed are a few examples of clients I'd just as soon forget, the "Craziest of the Crazies," who are some of the most unstable, offensive, and outright insane people I've ever met. If you're truly fortunate, your health club is devoid of people like this.

If not, know that I can relate to what you're going through – and that you have my deepest sympathies.

CALL 911!

Be it for a slip and fall, a training injury, or a cardiac arrest (I've done CPR more than once), the need to call 911 is pretty much inevitable.

During my years in the industry I witnessed hundreds of injuries – ranging in severity from "I need a Band-Aid" to "Oh God, I'm gonna die!" The worst were usually caused by accidents (machines breaking, cables snapping, etc.), but the majority were the result of good ol' fashioned stupidity.

Many guys got hurt doing what's known as "the Owl." While walking toward the steps leading to the gym floor, they'd see some scantily clad hottie riding the elliptical machine like it was a thrice-rescheduled conjugal visit.

Completely engrossed, they'd keep on walking, necks twisting almost to the breaking point, until they took a header right down the stairs.

At Caveat Sports, a girl once tripped on a sharp piece of metal that had been sticking out from under the edge of the steps. It caught on her sneaker and sent her tumbling headfirst down the stairs; she gashed open her head and lacerated her knee. When I wrote the accident report, my supervisor flipped out because, alas, I'd written down what actually happened. He promptly amended my report, and as you've undoubtedly guessed, they fixed those stairs *real* quick.

A similar thing happened twice at Empirical Sports, once to a delivery guy and again to the manager's daughter. Both times, I had to hold pressure bandages on their torn-open insteps while waiting for an ambulance.

A Chinese delivery guy was walking down the stairs, distractedly counting his money, and failed to realize that the plate glass window he was heading for wasn't a door. He put his head right through it, cutting his face to the bone in several places and splitting his nose open as well. I treated his injuries (my shirt was so bloodied, I looked like a survivor of the OK Corral), and gave him a $20 tip because I felt bad.

I offered to provide him with a great attorney, but unfortunately the guy couldn't sue because he was an illegal. The next day, the company had hastily repaired the glass and plastered it with all sorts of advertisements and posters, apparently to make sure it didn't happen again.

Training injuries are much more common. One day, I spotted a new member doing incline benches with the manager. From the way the two of them were bantering back and forth, it was obvious they knew each other. Unfortunately, the newbie wasn't as familiar with the incline bench as he was with his training partner. While sliding a 45 lb. plate off the end of the Olympic bar, he neglected to keep his eye (and grip) on it. When the plate reached the bar's end it slipped right through his fingers and dropped like a guillotine blade. Before my eyes, it smashed clean through the bones of his foot.

Another guy, "John," was using one of our squat racks, when a gentleman on a rack to his left started removing the plates off his bar. As all the weight was stripped off the left side (a *major* no-no) the three 45 lb. plates still on the right caused the bar to catapult up off the rack and whip toward John like a giant baton. *Except this was a six-foot, solid-steel baton weighing 45 lbs., propelled by 135 lbs. of weight and multiplied by centrifugal force.* It smashed into the rack with enough force to drop a rhino and just missed John's head. The poor guy came within inches of having his skull crushed. He turned sheet white and staggered out of the gym, shaken to the core.

And he never came back.

Despite their dull edges, weights make excellent meat cleavers. During my years at Empirical Sports, I saw a half-dozen guys chop off their fingers, usually with the dumbbells. They'd slam them back on the rack, not noticing, say, a protruding bolt between the two racks. The bolt's edge, combined with the dumbbell's mass and velocity, would shear right through flesh and bone, leaving fingers dangling by scraps of skin or twitching on the floor below.

Not a pretty picture.

Other guys were victims of their own laziness. They'd throw dumbbells around their weight bench, just because they didn't feel like putting them back. Eventually, their hands would drop after a tough set and a dumbbell on the floor found its way between the plates of the one in their hand, smashing their fragile fingers and knuckles into pulp.

You don't need weights to get injured in a gym: sometimes all you need is a good, solid wall. When I was at Empirical Sports I witnessed a horrific racquetball injury. These two particular guys often cursed at one another while competing. Since my office was adjacent to the courts, I was forced to endure their anger-fueled repartee. Normally, this didn't bother me, unless I was trying to close a sale (a little difficult when someone is yelling '*Mother fucker!*' at the top of their lungs).

On this particular day, however, the guys were really loud. I'd already closed my door, much to the relief of the panicky young lady in my office. Suddenly, I heard the most God-awful curse, followed by blood-curdling screams. I shook my head, apologized to my client, and stormed out to give them a piece of my mind (not that I could spare it). As I looked down, I saw one of them holding his arm and shaking all over. He couldn't even talk. He'd gone for a wild shot and extended his free arm to absorb his momentum as he hit the wall. The bones in his forearm had snapped like toothpicks and his arm was hanging like a piece of rubber. I remember spouting, "Jesus! Uh . . . hang on, dude! I'll call 911!"

The only thing worse is actually watching it happen. I once saw two guys get badly hurt working on Empirical Sports' basketball court. They were twenty feet up, using a scaffolding to work on the ceiling lights. Unfortunately, they were too lazy to climb down and move the scaffolding from light to light; instead they bounced it up and down in order to "hop" it from place to place. Eventually, the joints loosened and the inevitable happened. The scaffolding collapsed with a thunderous roar, ending up like a pile of steel Popsicle sticks. One guy was taken down in the crash and was half-buried in the wreckage. The other grabbed onto a sliver of metal that hung from the ceiling. There was no way to help him and no time to call 911. I watched in perverse fascination as his grip gave out and he fell screaming to the floor. He landed on the pile of broken scaffolding next to his friend.

The worst injury I ever witnessed happened to a guy doing squats at Dinar Fitness. He was using one of their old-fashioned Smith machines. He wasn't a particularly big guy, but he'd loaded a tremendous amount of weight on it – over 500 lbs. A concerned trainer asked him twice if he wanted a spot, and both times he declined. As I looked on, he got under the bar and started his lift. His legs shook violently as he slowly bent his knees. Then there was a wet, cracking sound, reminiscent of a chicken bone breaking, and one of his legs snapped in half just below the knee. He crashed straight to the floor, the impact drowned out by his hysterical screams.

Hate to say it, but I heard a rumor that the poor guy got an audition as one of the dwarves in the "Lord of the Rings."

SURVIVAL TIP #25

Hopefully by now you've realized that gyms can be very dangerous places. If you're going to use equipment, particularly the free weights, get yourself some help first – especially if you're doing an exercise you're not familiar with. Also, be aware of your surroundings and what the people nearby are doing. Watch your fingers when you put plates back on weight trees and dumbbells back on racks. And keep an eye out for loose weight bars and dumbbells. If you trip on a weight bar or land on a dumbbell you'll find out iron is not very forgiving.

Last, but not least, use common sense. If you're a guy, that hot brunette a few yards away won't know the difference between 200 lbs. and 400 lbs. so there's no need to kill yourself lifting more than you can handle to impress her. Should you end up hurting yourself, you'll have plenty of time to kick yourself for being such a dim-witted horn-dog.

CRAZIEST OF THE CRAZIES: MAN OF 10,000 FACES

One man, "Jack Kenmore," had more personalities than an outhouse has flies. That being said, he was often the highlight of my day. Jack used to waltz around Empirical Sports, having in-depth conversations with his many invisible friends. He must have been popular, because he knew more "people" than I could count. Some seemed more like enemies, though, because he and his unseen companions often got into very hostile verbal disputes.

I remember the first time I noticed Jack's abnormal behavior. He was riding a stationary bike and talking on the phone, trying to console someone whose sister just passed away. Then, as I walked by, I noticed something odd: Jack didn't have a phone – he wasn't even wearing a Bluetooth.

After that I paid much closer attention. Once, he sat on the end of a bench on the gym floor, pulled out a (real – not imaginary) clipboard and writing pad, and started hosting a corporate meeting. From what I could "see," at least two other people were involved in this meeting. Jack went back and forth between them, explaining their residuals and exit strategies. I'm not a corporate type, but it sounded very believable – his imaginary board members certainly knew their stuff. I walked away wondering if the stocks he'd mentioned were worth investing in, and whether it would count as some form of supernatural insider-trading.

Jack was married (a pharmacist client told me his wife came in weekly to pick up his assorted anti-psychotics), but his dress, mannerisms, and comments were undoubtedly gay. I don't know many gay men, and even fewer insane ones, but Jack's sexuality certainly spiced up his ghostly conversations.

One day, while passing through the men's locker room, I spotted Jack at a urinal. No one else was around. Suddenly, he started arguing with someone. His voice rose as he yelled, "Just *stop* it! It's *my* turn to shake it. You shook it *last* time!"

When I realized he was talking about his penis it was time to make myself scarce.

Another time, Jack got very agitated on a treadmill. Whoever he was talking to was upsetting him. Out of nowhere he snapped at his invisible friend, "No, you *can't* touch it. I don't *want* you to touch it! My penis is *fine*, thank you very much."

Editor's Note: Keep in mind that each of Jack's sentences is followed by a pause as he listens to the "response" of whoever is (supposedly) there.

Since I'd already heard Jack's Woody Woodpecker routine, and since we weren't in the locker room, I figured it was safe to go on eavesdropping. He continued his conversation with, "Look, I don't *care* what anyone says. 98.9% of the time I am completely happy with the size of my penis!"

I couldn't help but wonder what happened the other 1.1% of the time.

As a lark, I tried to coax my front desk staff into asking Jack for guest fees (It seemed appropriate for us to charge his "friend" for the day). I'd beg them, "Look, it's easy. All you have to do is say, 'Hey Jack, you got a pass for your friend?' and that's it!"

No one would do it. A few of the tougher guys *said* they would, but when the moment of truth came, they all chickened out. I can't say I blame them – crazy people are frightening. It's like in prison: the only people the really dangerous convicts fear are the lunatics. Nothing scares them. If they come after you, you have to kill them.

I finally had to do it myself (sort of).

We were having a fire drill, and I had to make sure all the members had left the club. As was typical, a few knuckleheads in the free weight area refused to put down their precious dumbbells and had to be "encouraged" to leave. I was overlooking the gym floor from upstairs and saw them lurking off to one side. Jack was nearby, wandering to and fro while talking to himself.

I shouted, "C'mon guys, let's go . . . everybody out!" I caught Jack's eye and added, "That means you, too, Jack! And bring your friends *with* you!"

There was a moment of hesitation as Jack glared up at me. Then his head lurched back and his eyes grew wild and furtive. His expression seemed to say, "Oh my God! He sees them *too!*"

One day, I had a bizarre conversation with Jack over the phone. He had a PIF (paid-in-full) membership, but one year he was short on cash. Maybe his wife spent his disability checks; in any case, he couldn't come up with the green. To help him out, I gave him a two week pass – with the understanding that he'd pay up when it ended.

Seventeen days later, Jack was MIA. I decided it was time to follow up and called his house. I knew his voice; after all, he'd been my client for a decade. Our conversation went like this:

"Hello?"

"Hi, Jack?"

"Who's calling?" Jack asked.

"It's Max from Empirical Sports."

All of a sudden, Jack's voice became soft and feminine. "Uh . . . this is his *mother*. Let me see if he's here."

Have you ever had a phone conversation where someone said something so bizarre that you found yourself holding the receiver and staring at it as if it just transformed into a live snake?

This was one of those times.

Adding to the weirdness was the fact that Jack's mother had passed away years prior. Images of Norman Bates and basements piled high with desiccated corpses filled my head. I nervously raised the receiver back to my ear and heard Jack's "mother" lower her voice and say, "It's Max from Empirical Sports."

Jack replied (in his own voice), "Oh crap!"

At this point I got pissed. I'm not usually aggressive with clients, but I absolutely *hate* when people bullshit me when I'm trying to help them out, no matter how psychotic they may be. As soon as "Jack" got back on the phone I laid into him.

"Don't you 'oh crap' me," I snapped. "I gave you two weeks free so you could come up with your renewal. It's been two and a half and you're nowhere to be found. Now get your ass in here!"

Jack became very flustered and apologized profusely. He swore on a stack of bibles he'd go to the bank and bring his renewal dues within the hour. And to my amazement, he did.

I guess even *crazy* people are afraid of pushy sales guys.

NOT SO SAFE

We've already covered the perils of locker robberies. But it should be pointed out that even club *safes* aren't impregnable. This matters a great deal to members who make cash payments for their monthly dues and PT packages without bothering to get a receipt – a bad move if that cash vanishes. And it often does. During my tenure at Empirical Sports, the club's safe was violated many times. Sometimes it was an outside job.

And sometimes it wasn't.

The first time the safe got hit I inadvertently saw the perpetrator casing the damn thing ahead of time. My manager, Antonia, was on her knees behind the front desk, fumbling with the safe's combination. As she did so, I noticed the front desk girl standing nearby, staring down at the safe's dial. I remember thinking, *She's not actually trying to memorize the combination, is she?*

I dismissed my suspicions as wanton paranoia – that is, until the following morning, when I found out that $1,800 in cash had vanished from the safe overnight. I immediately told Antonia what I'd seen, but it turned out to be unnecessary. Our resident safecracker and her partner in crime (another front desk associate) had bragged to some of their coworkers about their "big score" – not a smart move.

They were terminated the moment they walked back in the door.

Outside jobs were a lot more common. Burglars would break into the gym late at night, often by prying open a side door with a crowbar. They'd smash their way into offices through the drywall, raid the cash register, and steal whatever they could find. But it was always a waste of time: any cash still in the register was put in the safe at the end of each shift. And even if the burglars had a disgruntled associate who knew the safe combination, it would get them nowhere – the manager changed the combination every time someone who knew it was fired.

At least the thieves were usually smart enough to take the video tape out of the security system on their way out. I often marveled that, regardless of how much swag they managed to cart out of the place, they always got away before the cops responded to the burglar alarm.

I could expect crimes to be committed by disgruntled ex-members or ambitious receptionists. But I found that the most extreme theft was accomplished by a General Manager.

The "withdrawal" took place during a transition period between two club managers. The outgoing manager had a bad habit of leaving club cash in the safe for months on end, allowing it to accumulate into many thousands of dollars. He said it reduced his number of trips to the bank, but I suspect he "borrowed" cash from time to time and then replaced it before he made his deposits.

Whatever the case, the incoming manager discovered a ton of bread in the safe. He did a quick count and discovered there was over $10,000. That number didn't seem so large, however, when he checked the receipts and found out there was supposed to be at least *$15,000*. He immediately brought this up to his superiors and requested an audit for the following day, with another manager present. That night, a mysterious thief (who happened to have the club keys, alarm codes, and knowledge of the new digital security system) came into the club and emptied the safe of its contents.

I called my boss that following morning and he was flabbergasted when I told him what had happened. Even more so when I told him that corporate had named him as their primary suspect. After that, he disappeared without a trace, and I never heard from him again. The club's Assistant Manager (who had bridged the gap between the two managers) was fired on suspicion a few weeks later, and the original manager resigned shortly thereafter.

In the end, despite a boatload of finger pointing, no one took the rap. Some people thought that all three of them were involved, but that made no sense to me. Maybe if it was a few hundred grand, but I can't picture the three of them lying around sipping umbrella drinks in Fiji with only ten Gs between them.

CRAZIEST OF THE CRAZIES: THE COCKROACH

You don't have to bring cash or leave your wallet in your locker in order to get robbed. One locker room attendant at Empirical Sports had a sneakier way to take your money.

The "Cockroach" (or "Roach" for short) was many things: a thief, con man, and pervert. His grandiose schemes went far beyond pilfering cash and watches from lockers. When that wasn't enough, he tried his hand at identity theft.

It was my fault Roach got away with it . . . at least for a while. I gave him the info he needed, and I didn't even know it. When I signed up clients by phone, I wrote down their information on a piece of paper before putting it in the computer. Sometimes our network crashed and any on-screen info was lost, so rather than call a prospect back and ask them again (and look like an idiot), I'd write it down. Afterward, I simply crumpled up the paper and tossed it in the trash.

All of a sudden, someone started spending money on my client's credit cards. And no one could figure out how it was happening. They were being charged for computers, lap tops, online purchases – and the cards were still in their wallets. One client told me the chicanery started less than an *hour* after he signed up by phone, and the only thing he'd ever used his brand-new card for was the gym.

That was when I figured it out.

Roach had come across one of my cheat sheets while emptying my garbage and gave the credit card info to some of his less-than-honest friends. I should have realized something was amiss when he started constantly offering to empty my trash can. His area of responsibility was the men's locker room, and he wasn't exactly known for doing extra work. When I remembered that Roach had come by my office a half hour before my client called, I realized what was going on.

I was stunned and mortified. I reported the situation to my manager and admitted that I was partially responsible. Without any hard evidence, it was hard for Bates to do anything, so he cut open Roach's staff locker later that night.

The contents showed just how much of a con man he really was.

He had a slew of lockers downstairs, all securely padlocked. Inside we found huge stashes of contraband: jewelry, IPods, marijuana, condoms, lubricant, stacks of XXX magazines and DVDs, and enough liquor to throw a New Year's Eve party. Roach was running his own little bootleg business right out of the locker-room, pimping drinks to all the old-timers. He was their bartender and more, serving up booze, smokes, porn – you name it.

Needless to say, the contraband alone was grounds for immediate termination; they fired him post haste. And our members' credit card woes disappeared with him.

I can't say I was sorry to see the guy go. Even before we discovered his embezzlements, Roach had made quite a reputation by going around the gym and bragging about the size of his manhood. One day, my colleague Lance went up to him and flat-out asked, "I hear you got a huge cock. Is that true?"

Roach replied. "Yeah, but it's really curved when it's hard, so a lot of girls don't like it."

A few days later, Roach's curvy member made an appearance. He'd been hitting on our young Jamaican receptionist for weeks without success. Frustrated, he caught her alone in the parking lot and took matters "into his own hands."

Thankfully, I didn't witness this firsthand; all I know is the terrified girl came running into my office. Gasping for air, she told me Roach had approached her as she was exiting her vehicle and whipped his dick out. She told me (direct quote): "It was big and scabby and looked like the letter 'C'!"

Based on Lance's report, I knew she was telling the truth.

Unfortunately, the girl didn't testify, so he got away with it.

Appalling as this was, the Cockroach had far nastier habits – ones that made indecent exposure seem downright polite. A few weeks after the parking lot incident, he came into the manager's office and told us about his obsession with women's feces.

Yes, you read that right: *feces*.

Editor's Note: Just a friendly warning – anyone with gastric ulcers or a sensitive stomach might want to consider bypassing the next few pages. If not, don't say I didn't warn you.

Roach's greatest pleasure in life was having women shit on him; in fact, he lived for it. He liked to lie on the floor and have women squat down and take a steamy dump on his chest while he rubbed one out. And if they had diarrhea it was even better; he just put cellophane over his face so it didn't get in his eyes.

This was the guy cleaning the locker room, the steam room, the sauna, the showers . . .

Totally disgusted, I told Roach I'd had enough. Undeterred, he turned his attention to Bates, my manager, and enlightened him, in rich detail, about the contents of a woman's excrement – and his personal analysis of its scent, flavor, and consistency. He would take a woman's shit and smear it in his mustache so he could smell it throughout the day and think of her.

As I tried covering my ears, Roach opened his mouth and showed Bates where one of his molars was missing a huge filling. He said he'd take some crap and roll it between his fingers until it was a dried-up ball. Then he'd shove it inside his tooth like a replacement filling and suck on it throughout the day, savoring the flavor.

The last straw came when Roach suggested I try out his vile hobby. He suggested we put newspaper on my chest until I'd gotten used to the experience. My response can't be put into print – not even in *this* book.

"Man, you're just jealous because my dick's bigger than yours," he replied.

I smirked at him. "Well, I don't know about *that*, but I *do* know all about your 'letter C' problem, my friend. The front desk girl told us all about it. Unlike *you*, I don't need to have sex with women from around corners." I added some risqué pelvic motions to "drive my point home," and then added, "I'm a straight shooter, buddy. I *hit* what I aim at."

While Bates laughed uproariously, the Cockroach stormed red-faced out of the office. I guess I hit a sensitive spot, because he never spoke to me again.

Editor's Note: In retrospect, that was a very good thing, because I had run out of excuses for not shaking the guy's hand.

PARKING LOT PERILS

So, you've followed all my advice and left your club in one piece. Good job. You're home free now, right? Not so fast, pal. If your place has a parking lot, you still have one, final opportunity to experience some very nasty things.

Robberies and petty thefts don't just happen inside. Plenty of break-ins take place in the parking lots as well, which are often rife with thieves looking for an easy score.

Don't give them one.

Make sure your vehicle is locked up tight. Would-be entrepreneurs from seedy neighborhoods will sit in their car and study other vehicles, sometimes with binoculars, waiting for people foolish enough to leave a fancy purse or laptop in the backseat. They'll pull into an adjacent parking spot, smash a window, and then grab and go. Make sure valuables are stashed away from prying eyes; otherwise you're just asking for it.

Another thing: if you have a convertible, keep the top up. By showing that baby off to all the gym hotties and leaving it with the ragtop down, you're begging for problems. Thieves will steal anything they can pry loose, and an unexpected rainstorm is a *major* downer. I frequently paged members on the overhead to let them know their Benz was filling with water. It amazed me how quickly they'd sprint to the front desk.

They *never* ran that fast on the treadmill.

Besides break-ins, lots of other nasty things happen in gym parking lots – like drug dealing and prostitution. There's a seedy motel close by one of the Empirical Sports, and the hookers there worked it like you wouldn't believe.

They were incredibly ballsy. Sometimes they'd come ask to use the ladies room. The unspoken policy was to say "no," but one time a receptionist was stupid enough to say "yes," and allowed a scantily clad streetwalker inside.

A minute later, a woman came screaming out of the restroom because the hooker (I believe she called herself 'the Thunderbolt') was squatting in the sink in a reverse cowgirl position, rinsing out her genitalia.

Unpaid sex in gym parking lots is also very common, especially at night. Think about it: half-naked, pumped-up men and women who already have their juices flowing. Often they can't wait until they get home. Never mind the making out, the groping, and the occasional hummer – I walked out of Empirical Sports one night to find a hot, naked blonde in the backseat of a big SUV, sitting spoon-style on this guy's lap and riding him like Seabiscuit. This was thirty feet from our front door.

I couldn't help staring, partially because of the sight of her huge tits bouncing up and down, and partially because all the people passing by seemed completely unfazed.

Last but certainly not least, there's the violence. With all the testosterone, cheating, and adultery that go on, fighting is basically inevitable. I've broken up many serious weight-room brawls in my day, including one or two that could have been fatal.

And where do these guys go to resolve their beefs?

Outside.

SURVIVAL TIP #26

If cooler heads fail and there's a confrontation in the gym, look over your shoulder. There's nothing worse than getting clocked with a ten-pound plate in the middle of a set. And then there's your poor car to worry about. Vehicles are often vandalized in retaliation for some real or imagined slight. Key gouges, slashed tired, and broken lights, mirrors, and windshields were all common occurrences.

Remember, throwing fire on fire only makes things hotter. Throw water instead and even a juiced-up member will cool off. If you can't defuse things and shake hands, go find a manager. They can usually squash the conflict, especially when the respective parties are reminded that their memberships are on the line.

Remember: It's better to ask for help than to find yourself in trouble, or worse, needing to join another gym.

NEAR-FATAL ATTRACTION

You don't have to mess with muscleheads in order to put your life at risk. Sometimes all you have to do is just attract the wrong kind of woman.

"Kelly" was a tall, well-built babe who, at first glance, looked like a dream come true. At second glance, though, she was a walking nightmare. She had some serious issues, and the rest of the gym used to call her "Special K." Why? Because Kelly was the stalker from hell. After consummating a relationship with a man, she'd haunt him until the day he died.

It happened to my poor buddy "Sly." He dated her for a month and thought he was in hog heaven. Then one day they got into a huge fight (He made a joke about having a threesome with one of her girlfriends). Kelly had a unique way of expressing her displeasure – she blasted him in the jaw with a right cross that nearly knocked him cold.

Mind you, he was driving at the time.

Sly told me Kelly stalked him for *years*, despite a restraining order and rotating phone numbers. She'd bake him cookies and drop them off at his mom's house. She also followed him to nightclubs, usually in her pajamas, and would wait in her car until 4 a.m. so she could trail him to another girl's house and then start ringing the doorbell. And on other nights, she'd scale the fire escape across the street from his apartment and watch him while he slept using night vision binoculars.

No joke.

When I met Kelly, this knowledge was foremost on my mind.

I noticed her hanging out by the front desk. She looked distressed, so I took a chance and asked her what was wrong. She needed a ride home and asked if I'd drive her to Queens. I declined; I lived only four blocks away, and there was no *way* I was sitting for two hours in bumper-to-bumper traffic.

Hours later, Kelly was still forlornly sitting there. I felt bad and offered her a lift to the nearest car service. A few blocks away, I realized I hadn't eaten and asked if she minded me hitting up a fast food joint. She made a face and suggested "we" eat something healthier instead.

The next thing I knew, I was taking her to dinner.

We ended up in some halfway-decent Chinese restaurant. I noticed Kelly refused to sit with her back to the door (apparently she had a lot of enemies). While we ate she told me a charming story about her recent fight with a female bodybuilder over some guy. She'd yanked the girl out of her car window, wedged her under a wheel well, and stomped her leg until it broke in three places.

As I listened, I started scheming for ways to get the hell out of there. Especially when she started saying things like, "I don't understand why you work in the gym. You're so much *better* than those people." Knowing what she'd put my friend through, there was no way in *hell* I'd do anything with her.

I paid the check and we headed to the car. Kelly brought up that I lived only a few blocks away and suggested, "in the interest of convenience," that we go to my apartment and call her cab from there. I felt a sudden chill. I knew if I took her to my place she was going to be all over me.

Therein lay disaster.

As a compromise, I decided to call from the car and have the cabbie meet us. I started driving, all the while sweating bullets. A car service took usually fifteen minutes, sometimes twenty.

Those were the longest four blocks of my life. I felt like I was driving to the electric chair.

As we pulled up out front Kelly purred hotly in my ear. "Gee, the cab's not here. I guess we'll have to wait *inside*." As my butt cheeks tightened, I spotted a set of headlights in my mirror.

Gods be praised, my savior had arrived – and in record time!

I gave a huge sigh of relief and ejected myself from the car. "Your chariot awaits, my dear," I said.

Kelly got out, a look of disappointment on her face. "Oh well, your loss."

Before I could yelp, she grabbed me and shoved her tongue in my mouth. I held the cab door for her and sent her on her way.

I saw Kelly in the gym several times after that and not once did I mention our "dinner date," or be so insane as to ask for her number. One day, I overheard her gossiping with two of the receptionists. They were discussing the restaurants men took them to and how cheap guys were.

I chimed in, "When *I* take a girl out, she's lucky if she gets Chinese food."

Kelly gave me an unfriendly look. "That's why you and I never had a second date," she remarked.

"No, we never had a *first* date," I corrected her. "And if we *had* gone on a date, there *still* wouldn't have been a second one. Do you know why?"

"Why?"

"Because you *scare* me," I said. Trying not to look over my shoulder, I fled to my office – and contemplated bricking up the door.

SURVIVAL TIP #27

Be very selective when it comes to dating people in the gym. If something goes wrong (and it usually does), there will be no escaping them.

And forget just feeling uncomfortable. What if your ex is off balance? Twice after our last conversation, Kelly threw punches at me – haymakers, in fact. The first time we were in a restaurant next door, and the second time on the weight floor.

I was lucky. Both times I was able to put a barrier between us (tables and weight machines work great) until she calmed down. But it was an embarrassing recipe for disaster.

So, keep in mind, as great as that girl on the stepper might look – all covered with sweat, with that tight, perky butt of hers sticking way out – think twice before sticking your "neck" in her "noose."

You never know. Her name just might be Kelly!

CHAPTER 19:

BLOOD FROM A STONE

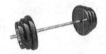

This chapter is primarily geared toward fellow gym rats and those interested in a fitness career. It exposes the innermost workings of gyms and how they treat (and mistreat) their respective sales staff.

After my final encounter with Empirical Sports' CEO Matt Jones, I was forced to accept that, to the people in charge, I, my coworkers, and all of my members, were just cogs in their monstrous, money-making machine. It was frightfully apparent from the way they treated their people and their scarily high turnover rate. I'd heard many in the industry say, "You're only as good as your last month." To an employer, the value of a sales rep is measured by comparing them to their last month's quota.

And it's true.

Fellow reps came and went, even the ones I liked. Sometimes they were fired for political reasons, sometimes they screwed up, but often as not they had simply gotten tired and let their numbers drop. Someone could be a top seller for years, but if they fell into a slump for more than a few *days* they became the weak link in the chain. At that point, they had to start watching their back.

Fitness companies are especially cold and mercenary towards their sales and management teams. At least 80% of their revenue comes from memberships, so they squeeze the sales staff to wring out every drop of profit. Employees feel like they're working in a giant pressure cooker and suffer from burn-out and exhaustion. When the dried-up husk of a sales rep or manager has nothing left to give, corporate just flings them away like a used condom and moves on to the next victim.

It's the truth.

CORPORATE CUTBACKS

You can always tell when a fitness company is struggling. If the company is publicly traded, like Empirical Sports or Caveat Sports, you pick up on it from the oh-so-slow death spiral their stock performs as shareholders watch their investments dissolve into nothingness. From the inside, though, the indications are subtler.

For members, their immediate concern is whether or not their club remains open. Stories abound of gyms closing up shop in the middle of the night and disappearing with all their equipment – and their clients' hard-earned cash.

Most health clubs are required by law to post a large bond as collateral in order to protect their members from just such an occurrence. They're also required to have copies of it on hand and available to be viewed upon request. If you have your doubts about a gym, don't hesitate to ask to see it.

I worked for Empirical Sports for many years, but as the economy took hit after hit, I saw trends that made me wonder how much longer I'd have a job. The first year I worked there we got a Christmas bonus. It wasn't much, a week's salary, but at least it was *something*.

The following year, I opened my holiday check and discovered they had replaced my bonus with some free movie tickets. Each and every one of us received complimentary tickets to the cinema. For the record, this was what's known as a barter deal. My employers didn't even pay for those "re-admission" tickets.

The next thing on the chopping block was our annual holiday party. The year after that, our movie tickets disappeared. Next went our corporate meetings. Normally, my company hosted their monthly meetings at a rented hall in the city. They switched to having them at a movie theater. Then, they had them broken down regionally and held at clubs in each respective area. Finally, they stopped the meetings altogether and converted them to more sensible (and cost-effective) conference calls.

Salary changes followed. During my initial years at Empirical Sports, sales reps were entitled to an annual raise of $1/hour. That added up to $40/week, or about $160/month. It wasn't much. After my manager informed me about my "big" dollar raise, I replied, "Wow, now I can buy that extra can of diet cola I've always wanted." Soon they chopped even that, reducing it to only fifty cents. Then, to top it off, I was informed that I was "capped" and couldn't even *receive* a raise. The last five years I worked there they never raised my salary a penny.

Looking back, I realized this salary cap wasn't just them being cheap. It was another indication of how short-term careers in fitness usually are. They don't expect someone to last more than five years, so there's no compensation plan in place for salespeople beyond that point.

When a company is really feeling the pinch, *no* area is safe. The next place to get bitten at my club was personal training. In the beginning, when a person joined they were given two one-hour sessions. This was reduced to a single, one-hour session, then that was cut to forty-five minutes, and then again to thirty. I was very concerned at that point.

How much can you possibly teach someone in half an hour?

Of course, the reason for hacking away at orientation sessions had nothing to do with paying trainers, who got paid minimum wage floor hours for doing them. It was to pressure members into shelling out for PT packages. When people realized they knew nothing about working out and their club wasn't going to give them instruction, they were much more inclined to purchase PT, thereby increasing ancillary revenue.

Editor's Note: The fitness companies' logic here is inescapable. If you owned a gym, would you rather have clients paying $75 per month or per hour?

The next indication of corporate belt-tightening came when they reduced our vacation time, sick days, and holidays. Most places made it difficult, if nigh impossible, to take a day off. If you were sick they made you jump through hoops: you had to call your club, your manager, and even your area manager to tell all of them you were ill. Some of that is understandable. But telling an employee that they can't take a sick day without finding coverage is unreasonable. Frankly, if I were in bed with a 103-degree fever, that's asking too much. You expect me to find a last-minute shift replacement while I'm busy dying?

Not going to happen.

The same thing applied to holidays and vacations. For a sales rep, taking a vacation was stressful enough, especially when you knew you'd be losing a grand or more in commissions while you were gone. To make matters worse, we were asked to secure coverage from another club for our week's shifts – a tactic designed to make vacations much more difficult. Just one more indicator of a company struggling to stay afloat in a downward-spiraling economy.

At one memorable meeting at Empirical Sports, they announced that our sick days and paid holidays were being abolished in favor of what they called Personal Time Off (PTO). The official idea was that employees were now getting "x" number of days off, based on tenure, and they could use them for whatever they saw fit: holidays, sick days, or personal days.

After doing some mental calculations, I realized we were being shortchanged in total days/hours. The company even stopped honoring national holidays. I had a lot of tenure already, but for the new guys it was a major shaft job.

I eventually found a silver lining and worked the PTO thing to my advantage. Having been there for many years, I was highly trusted by management. I was also a salaried employee and got set pay (sans commissions) for my workweek, regardless of overtime. I also was responsible for putting my hours in each week, which were then validated by my manager without a second thought.

I started to proactively put my hours in for a month in advance. Besides reducing my workload, this had an unexpected perk. After I took a sick day, I was often so besieged upon my return that I forgot to correct my hours for that day (i.e. change it to consume one of my PTO days). Since my overworked manager never remembered me being sick, I got an extra three or four days off each year.

The company was already making us work a twelve-hour shift on the last day of the month, even if it was the weekend (you didn't get paid for an extra day, nor was there any time-and-a-half for extra hours). Then they decided that for us to deserve a lunch break (which was mandated by law, and which they were "appalled" to discover many people hadn't been taking), we had to work nine hours instead of the traditional eight.

Editor's Note: The unwritten law in health clubs is that you don't take a lunch break. They expect you to eat at your desk and keep calling clients.

I crunched the numbers: by adding on this extra hour, Empirical Sports was basically hijacking 260 hours of our lives each year. That broke down to 6.5 *weeks* of free labor (at a rate of eight hours a day). Not surprisingly, people objected to this, including a few of their top managers and sales reps.

They were told to either deal with it or walk.

Then, adding insult to injury, someone at corporate came up with an even more novel idea. They decided all sales staff and managers should be required to work three of the last four days of each month, in addition to the last day's twelve-hour shift. Since I worked Monday to Friday, I was now getting screwed for an additional weekend day almost every month (again, without pay), *and* an extra three hours on top of my already extended shift.

At this point, I made sure that, whether it was that twelve-hour closeout shift, or one of those extra weekend days, I became terribly sick immediately afterward and used one of my PTO days. And I did it every time. No one ever seemed to notice that one of the company's top consultants kept calling in right after closeout, month after month and year after year.

I always wished they'd question me about it. I had a great song prepared about how exhausted I was from working so hard and how the long hours and endless stress had made my immune system collapse.

LET THEM EAT LATE . . .

Empirical Sports then held a surprise meeting where they unexpectedly announced a major change in their sales reps' schedules – and that they were "doing us a big favor." They'd decided that it was wrong that most of us worked until 9 p.m. or later each day. They wanted us to have a regular shift like most Americans, 9 a.m. to 6 p.m., so we could be home in time to have supper with our families. The announcement was met with jubilant cheers by just about everyone.

Everyone except me, that is.

I'd been around long enough to know that something else was going on. No health club chain does something like that unless there's something in it for them. Calling it a "favor" was fluff designed to keep people from discerning the company's real agenda. I sat there, listening attentively, and waiting for the other shoe to drop.

My wait was not a long one.

We were expected to go out like gangbusters and sell-sell-sell, then head home by 6 p.m. to enjoy the fruits of our well-deserved labors. On the surface it sounded all well and good, but the fine print stated that we were still responsible for our sales quotas. And anyone who's worked in fitness knows that 2/3 of the business walks in the door between 5 and 9 p.m., including most of your scheduled appointments. So how were we supposed to hit our numbers?

We weren't.

The company expected their entire sales force to falter and realize they were in danger of losing their jobs. To avoid termination, they'd start putting in extra hours and stay late, probably 8 or 9 p.m. as usual. The company's executives were herding their sales reps and managers into working a 9 to 9 day – a Caveat Sports trademark. They wanted to turn their employees into indentured servants, making them work sixty-hour shifts instead of the forty-five they were already doing, while paying them for only forty. Once people got acclimated to this form of servitude, they'd make it the norm and new employees would *have* to put in those hours.

Fortunately, their plan backfired.

They miscalculated how much fear they generated, and how team-oriented their people really were. Like most of my colleagues, I put in my required 9-6 shift and then strutted out the door without a care in the world. I wouldn't stay late for anything, and there was nothing they could do about it; I was still hitting my quota. Sure, I wasn't burying it like I normally would have, and I had to work harder in order to hit, but as long as my numbers were there I was untouchable.

The other sale reps weren't doing so well, however, and the company's numbers rapidly plummeted. After some anonymous letters were sent to the major papers and the USDOL that exposed the company's ongoing labor-related shenanigans, the company must have been inspired to take action. A few months later, our old shifts were quietly reinstated and no one ever said why.

I wonder who sent those letters.

UNDER THE MICROSCOPE

Many chains use their appointment books in order to wring additional hours from their staff.

At Empirical Sports, we were given a new book each month. Inside we were asked to list our "required quota," as well as our "desired goal," which was supposed to be substantially higher. At that point our quotas meant nothing; whatever we put in for our desired goal was what the company would hold us accountable for. Rebel that I was, I always kept my quota and goal the same, much to my superiors' annoyance.

There were also positive and negative sections to the planner. In the positive section, known as the "benefits" part, we were instructed to list the rewards we'd reap from meeting and exceeding our self-inflated quotas. They expected us to write things down like, "buy a new car" or "make a down payment on a house." This section was ultimately there to mentally offset the negative portion, also known as the "consequences" section.

This was what the company *really* wanted us to fill out. They wanted us to write down what we were prepared to do if it looked like we weren't going to hit our numbers. We were *encouraged* to write things like: "I'll put in extra hours each day" and "I'll come in on my days off." We were supposed to sign off on whatever we wrote down, with the manager co-signing to witness it.

Basically, the company asked us to make ourselves slaves. By writing down and signing off on what they wanted – giving the company grounds to fire us, should we fall short of our obligations – we were committed to work extra days and hours, and all without pay. And, as mind-boggling as it was to me, they expected us to agree to it with no questions asked.

For seven years they tried getting me to put my neck in that noose, and each and every time I declined. They pressured me, threatened me, and told me every other salesperson in the company had done it, but I steadfastly refused to be one of them. I may not be the sharpest tool in the shed, but I ain't the dullest either.

Things got even worse after Empirical Sports stopped doing TV ads. Instead of spending money to build their business, their corporate bigwigs decided that money was put to better use in their pockets. They put the responsibility of driving business squarely on the collective shoulders of their already beleaguered salespeople. Their reps would now go door-to-door, like traveling salesmen, and magically create interest in unwary people so they'd come in and join.

We were supposed to speak to dozens people each day and solicit appointments. It didn't matter *where* these people came from, we had to do it and that was that. As an added motivator, the manager was supposed to call and *confirm* our appointments in order to make sure they were genuine.

Editor's Note: Only occasionally did this make sense. I remember seeing one of my peers' appointment books; in it, he had appointments with both Hulk Hogan and Evander Holyfield (amazingly, neither showed up). For the most part, though, having your boss call your already-scheduled clients is the world's stupidest idea. It's like having your dad phone a girl twice before your first date, just to make sure you were still on; it reeks of desperation.

If we didn't come up with our minimum number of appointments, we were then punished by being taken off the "up-system" and could no longer pitch to guests and walk-ins.

I always hated the term "walk-in," especially if my front desk staff would introduce a potential client by saying, "He's a walk-in." It made my customers feel dehumanized, like they were nothing more than a number on someone's bottom line. I'd correct my co-worker by saying, "No, he's not. What you mean is he's interested in *membership*."

The new sales system was doomed to die, but there was no point in sharing my opinion. I'd be branded a poor team player. Besides, I knew from painful experience that no one would listen anyway. To them, I was just some schmuck who consistently signed up a thousand people a year. What could I possibly know?

Although Caveat Sports is awful, the one smart thing they do is advertise. They *have* to; it offsets their less-than-sterling reputation and also makes their clubs look damn good on TV. By using the power of television to show off sexy, shapely bodies, they generate interest. Their phones are dead all day until those commercials hit. *Then* their lines light up. I was there and I know.

It's all about sparking interest.

Seven out of eight people who join health clubs either walk in the door or call first to make an appointment. The remainders are mostly referrals from the gym's existing member base. That's how it is, and anyone who can't understand that is in the wrong line of work. Yes, it's good for you, but working out is hard work. And it takes a serious amount of interest to get someone to come down to a gym and sign up. You're not going to grab some girl off the subway and hypnotize her into joining. People need a powerful, burgeoning need before they're willing to make a major investment of their time and money. Sure, you might get lucky and happen upon someone who's already there mentally, but that's a rarity. Like I said before, people want to go about their lives without being bothered by pushy salespeople. Don't you?

Hell-bent on their new sales system, however, Empirical Sports began doing something every employee loves – micro-managing their people. They started a system of checks and balances; besides our day planners we were handed monthly appointment planners to list and update our pending clients for weeks in advance.

Then we were given the dreaded "Primary Incoming Scheduled Sales" book.

The PISS book was a big binder at the front desk, wherein we *again* listed all of our appointments, and their contact numbers, so the manager could call and confirm them. Then, on top of *that*, we were handed plastic boxes with dividers for every day of that month. We were supposed to fill them with the tour cards of any clients that didn't join, so we could follow up with them when appropriate.

The depressing thing was that our regular planners already had all of this information, and the manager could see it at any time. In fact, they *did* see our books – every day. But that was the way the company wanted it. So we spent a huge chunk of our day writing the same info over and over again, just to justify their sales system. It would have made more sense to spend that time calling clients or bonding with members.

If there was ever a shred of doubt in my mind about how my employers viewed their sales reps, it was whisked away the day I walked into my manager's office. She was on a conference call and listening to some company big shot preaching about how the managers were to motivate their sales teams. His spiel was, "Each of your sales people should have at least four new appointments and two 'drag-ins' by 9 a.m. each day. We want at least four call drives per day – an hour each. And you should be in there while they make those calls. Stand behind them and pace back and forth to create a sense of urgency. And stay on top of your people. If you see a salesperson without a phone in their ear, get the duct tape!"

In case that didn't make sense, by 9 a.m. (precisely when your shift started) you were supposed to have already magically made four new appointments (maybe by calling from home?) *and* you were supposed to find two poor people while on your way to work (i.e. someone who took the train with you or was biking by where you parked your car) and physically drag them into the club.

I can't see the motivational benefit of looming over someone while they called potential customers. I *hate* having someone in the room with me while I'm on the phone. It makes a lot of salespeople nervous, eliminates any chance at a personal approach, and it's a major invasion of privacy. Not to mention it cuts down on their ability to close appointments.

If my any of my bosses tried that with me, I'd have politely told them, "Get the %#@*! out of my office."

Come to think of it, they *did* try it, and I *have* done exactly that, more than once . . .

GIVE ME YOUR TIRED, YOUR POOR, AND YOUR FRIENDS TOO!

People are most likely to refer others to their gym during the first few weeks after joining. They're so excited about the place that they want their friends to join too – there's strength-in-numbers.

My company capitalized on this by squeezing anything they could out of each new client, starting the moment they joined. One way was via their "friendly referral" promotion. Once your contract was printed, you were asked to fill out a form with the names, addresses, and numbers of your closest friends and relatives. You'd be told, "Normally our guest fee is $20.00 per day, but right now you can receive free one-week trial memberships for all your friends and family members. Just fill this out while I get your paperwork together, and I'll be right back."

Naturally, people were reluctant to throw their friends under the bus. So the sales team was trained to apply pressure: "You don't want to work out alone, do you? Who's your best friend? Would they like to work out with you? Who else do you know who needs to lose weight or get healthier? What about your family? Are they excited about training too? Let's get them down here to support you!"

In the end, it was just a profit-motivated tactic to turn one sale into three. You can't blame a company for trying to milk the cow, but don't tear the poor thing's udders off!

Personally, I never used the "referral at point of sale" technique. I thought it was greedy and grasping, not to mention pathetically transparent. Of course, it was company policy, so I always jotted down that I'd gotten one or two referrals from every new client. It was nonsense, but I was good at my job, so my managers never bothered confirming it. They all knew I was faking it; they just didn't want to ruffle the goose laying all those golden eggs. Why fix something that isn't broken?

I personally never needed corporate head games in order to be successful. I got plenty of referrals from my people; I just never had to ask for them. And *that* is the secret to being a great salesperson. There were hundreds of times when a member walked in with a friend in tow, looking for me to sign them up. If I wasn't there, they'd ask when I would be, then turn around and leave. And they'd reject any of my competitors, looking to hog in on my action.

Once day, I witnessed this first hand. One of my guys stalked into the lobby with his friend. Not realizing I was in my boss's office, he breezed past the front desk, ignoring the receptionist's attempts to stop him, and looked for me in my office. He then turned to my front desk girl and asked, "Where's Max?" Before she could utter a reply, he held up a hand.

"My boy's here to join and he ain't seeing nobody but Max, so don't try handing us over to one of your bullshit sales guys. You got me?"

Of course, I walked right over to set things right, but this happened constantly. Many times my boss approached my clients and offered to sign up their referral. Each time they told her, "Go back to your office." She thought it was scary and wondered what I did to instill such maniacal loyalty in my clients.

Truth is, there wasn't much to tell. It was a simple combination of good personality and taking care of your people. When my clients realized I had their best interests at heart, they'd do just about anything for me. They brought me gifts, sent me drinks in clubs, and picked up my tab in restaurants. One time, a client even offered to beat the snot out of someone they thought was being rude to me.

Thankfully, I resisted the urge to take them up on such a tempting offer.

SURVIVAL TIP #28

If a gym sales rep is pressuring you into giving referrals, make sure you text your friends for permission before giving out any of their personal information. Nothing spoils a friendship faster than feeding your buddy to an avaricious salesman – you wouldn't want it done to you.

Resist the pressure. Ask your sales rep for guest passes instead. If that fails, and you absolutely can't get out of it, give out just their email addresses. Unlike an in-your-face salesman, you can eliminate them with the push of a button.

CHAPTER 20:
MY GYM, MY PHARMACY

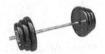

Any story of the fitness industry would be incomplete without airing out the dirtiest laundry. It's something you'll never read about in any aerobics class schedule or mission statement: the rampant use of drugs.

Drug dealing, and the side effects their non-prescribed usage often precipitates, takes place in just about every health club in the country. It happens in the parking lot, in the locker room, in storage areas, and even in the offices. The frequency might vary from location to location, but trust me – it's common no matter where you go. Whether it's the sale of dangerous anabolic steroids or more "harmless" recreational drugs like marijuana and cocaine, it's there if you know where to look.

I guarantee it.

JUICE ON THE LOOSE

Forget what you heard from that "innocent" salesperson, because the use and sale of anabolic steroids happens in practically every weight facility in the *world* – certainly in every one I ever worked. Trafficking in steroids is against the law (a felony, to be precise), but it's a big business for gym rats looking to make a quick buck. At serious bodybuilding gyms, experienced dealers lurk in every corner.

I can vouch for this via personal experience. I was twenty-four years old the first time I was pitched steroids. I'd been training for six years and had gone from a scrawny 130 lbs to a rock-hard and athletic 190. I looked good, the women in my life loved me – but I just wasn't satisfied. I wanted to be like the Greek gods I saw swaggering around my gym. I wanted "big guns," a 500 lb. bench press, and the power and presence to go up on a bodybuilding stage and blow my opponents away from the sheer shock wave brought on by my poses.

It became apparent to me, however, that I had hit a plateau and would never achieve my goal.

That's when the pusher came at me.

Steroid distributors are just like any other opportunistic drug dealers. I was a young guy frustrated beyond belief – the perfect target. I remember "Mike's" sales pitch to this day: "We can give you something that will give you more gains in the next month than you'll see in the next two years."

"You mean steroids?"

"Yep."

"But I heard they're bad for you. And don't you lose everything you gain once you stop taking them?"

"They're only bad if you don't know what you're doing. And we'll give you stuff to take so you don't lose anything."

And *that's* how I got sucked in.

As I found out, there *is* no drug that will maintain your "ill-gotten" gains: it was just his ploy to get me hooked. But I didn't know that at the time.

Steroid usage is intoxicating. Your testosterone levels soar and you feel invincible – like you can turn over a truck. Every day you see and feel yourself getting bigger and stronger. I gained 20 lbs in a month. If I hadn't blown out my shoulder trying to lift too much weight (and been forced to stop training for two months), I might have become a lifelong addict. Luckily, that mandatory respite and detox helped me clear my head. I told Mike and his supplier to stick their pills where the sun doesn't shine and never looked back.

I will tell you, however – in purely clinical terms – that while I was on "the shit" I was one *nasty* motherfucker. I was moodier than a wolverine with PMS, and my already-short temper turned completely vicious at the drop of a hat (which explains why there's so much violence in gyms – something we'll touch on momentarily).

The "juice" is everywhere, not just in professional sports. One Empirical Sports Club seemed perfectly corporate and professional . . . until the day when all the men's room toilets were clogged. It was so bad they had to bring in a plumber. When he finally discovered the source of the problem, he had the manager go down there because he couldn't believe what he'd found. The traps under the toilets were completely jammed up – with over a *thousand* hypodermic needles.

It turned out that members were flushing their used needles down the toilet after shooting up in the stalls.

Every gym I worked at had steroid dealers, but the managers never seemed to do anything about it. All you had to do was to train there for a few weeks until you had a familiar face, and then ask the bigger guys where they got their stuff. It's easy to tell who is on the juice, and there are many signs besides sheer size. Excessive use makes your skin change; it becomes puffy and often takes on a reddish or pinkish hue. Juiceheads may have unnaturally low body fat levels, out-of-control acne, hair loss, and an irascible disposition.

Women who take steroids also become extremely muscular. They lose their breasts, grow heavy, angular jaws, and their voices deepen (think butch drag queen). And *anyone*, male or female, who takes Human Growth Hormone (HGH) ends up with even more pronounced (and permanent) side effects. Their hands and feet elongate, and their jaw and brow ridges grow thicker and more pronounced. Real Herman Munster stuff.

Makes you wanna run for that needle, doesn't it?

For sure, once you discover who the dealers are and gain their confidence, you can pretty much get anything you want: Dianabol, Methyl testosterone, Deca durabolin, Anadrol-50 . . . you name it. As long as you have the cash and can keep your mouth shut, you too can become a pharmaceutically enhanced freak.

Over time, I discovered that not only my members were pushing this poison. Many of the trainers I knew (including the women) weren't just taking steroids – they were selling them, too. One General Manager at Empirical Sports actually sold Russian Dianabol (also known as D-bol) and HGH out of his back office, right there in the lobby.

How do I know about this?

Because the maniac proudly showed me his stash, piled up neatly on his office desk, and then tried selling me some!

Steroid use has inherent health risks and side effects. They are addictive and can potentially kill. They do horrific damage to your internal organs, especially your liver, and cause things other than muscle to grow in your body, like *tumors*. After just a month of taking Anadrol-50 I had an enlarged liver. A few years later, I developed cysts on one of my kidneys and had to have a tumor the size of a softball removed from my throat.

I'm fine now, thank God. But others weren't so lucky.

I lost many clients and friends. One guy was napping on his sofa when his liver ruptured, killing him in his sleep. His poor wife came home and found him lying there, dead. Another guy dropped dead in his kitchen of a massive heart attack. And he was alone with his toddler at the time. Can you imagine what his family went through, especially that innocent little kid?

SURVIVAL TIP #29

I don't care how eager you are to get in shape, or how tempting it is to cut corners. Do yourself a favor and leave the juice for the juice-heads. There's a popular saying in the gym: "Keep taking steroids and you'll be the biggest man in the cemetery." And graveyards aren't exactly popular pick-up spots . . .

BAD BLOOD

Steroid-induced violence happens a lot, especially in the smaller, less cosmopolitan places that cater to your average Joe. It's also more common among men, who tend to use steroids more frequently. I've witnessed verbal disputes, one-on-one scuffles between rival males, and an all-out brawl that took a riot squad to break up. I've also confronted dozens of juiced-up muscleheads over the years.

Fortunately, I almost always managed to keep my temper in check.

Others are not so reserved.

When I was at Empirical Sports, one of my oversized managers got into a fistfight right in his office. His opponent was "Biff," a neighborhood hooligan (and consummate steroid user) who'd been using the place for free by giving his friend's name. One day, the receptionist caught on and told her boss. He confronted Biff and told him to either buy a membership, or leave and not come back. Our "guest" replied, "Go fuck yourself. I'm not paying, and I'm gonna *keep* using the gym. And there's *nothing* you can do about it."

Quick as a cat, the manager blasted Biff in the jaw, knocking him out cold with one punch. Then, he dragged him outside and deposited him in the dumpster to be picked up with the trash.

I guess Biff didn't expect such attentive customer service.

I broke up a steroid related fight myself soon after. I was doing a post-work-out stretch when two big goons started *killing* each other just a few yards away. I had my headphones on, so at first didn't even know a fight had broken out until I noticed a ring of cheering guys some fifty feet away. In the middle of this surging sea of testosterone, two lifters were ferociously slugging it out.

At first, I thought they were just clowning around, but I quickly realized I was wrong. They must have been brawling for a while; they were both soaked with sweat and completely out of breath. Fatigue meant nothing to them; when they reached the point of exhaustion, they'd back up, suck in a few desperate breaths, and then charge in again, fists flailing. Forty people stood there watching this – including one of my personal trainers – and no one was doing a damn thing. It was like something out of "Fight Club."

I dropped my headphones and bowled over a half dozen guys as I burst through the crowd. In seconds I was between two battling brown bears – and struggling to wrench them apart (Looking back, I have no idea *what* I was thinking).

As my two would-be combatants surged at one another, I bellowed at them to, "cut the shit and take it outside," or else forfeit both their member-ships. I also reamed out my PT, who remained ringside the entire time, his arms folded across his chest as he eagerly watched the battle.

I eventually restored order and found out what caused the fight. Apparently, they were both dealing steroids. "Scrugg" discovered that "Bruiser" had tried to break into his house a week earlier and steal his inventory, and Scrugg had been gunning for him ever since. He even told me that he'd lain in wait for Bruiser outside the locker rooms with a 10 lb. dumbbell in hand, hoping to bash him over the skull with it.

Unfortunately, Bruiser got wind of the ambush and snuck out the back door. Not willing to lose his last opportunity for revenge, Scrugg caught up and sucker-punched him.

The most epic steroid-fueled brawl took place at an Empirical Sports in Brooklyn between an ex-cop, and, ironically enough, an ex-convict. As a re-sult of my position I knew that "Paul" and "Jackie" were both serious weight-lifters who regularly enjoyed their "pharmaceutical delights."

I also knew there was a lot of bad blood between them.

I don't know exactly what started the fight, although I heard afterward that one of them owed the other a ton of cash from a drug deal. What I *do* know is that, out of nowhere, Jackie went charging at Paul (who was in the middle of a set of barbell curls) and screamed, "You motherfucker!" before blasting him hard in the temple. Paul shrugged it off, and the two then grappled like a pair of rabid pit-bulls, punching, biting and eye gouging each other while a half-dozen guys struggled to break it up.

There was no stopping them. They were so big and strong and filled with rage that no one could do anything. When their fists failed to inflict enough damage, they started hitting each other with weight bars and Olympic plates. Desperate calls were made to the police. By the time the fight ended, the place looked like a demilitarized zone. Twenty cops had taken over the gym floor, and blood was spattered on a half-dozen weight machines.

After the fight, Paul remained upstairs, talking to a few on-duty cops, while Jackie hid out downstairs in the locker room (He eventually snuck out the back to avoid arrest). Paul eventually told me that he needed to go downstairs to get stuff from his locker. To prevent the start of round seven, I offered to go get his stuff for him.

As I walked into the locker room I found Jackie stalking back and forth. He was bruised and bloodied and shaking with rage, while a friend of his desperately tried to calm him down. I'd never seen a real "roid rage" before, but I have to tell you, it was damn scary. Jackie spotted me and roared, "*You!* You're his *friend!*"

The next thing I knew, a 250 lb. maniac was charging at me with drool running down his chin and murder in his eyes. I can usually take care of myself, but I'd had shoulder surgery three weeks prior and my right arm was still in a sling, so I wasn't too thrilled with the idea of taking him on.

To my astonishment, Jackie's burly friend grabbed him in mid-charge and hoisted him bodily into the air, slamming him like a rag doll against a nearby locker. He held him there, and bellowed, "*Now* what the fuck are you doing? The kid didn't do anything to you!"

Jackie's mad-dog eyes rolled wildly around until they gradually came into focus. I don't know if whatever he was on had worn off, but he looked at me in confusion. "He's right . . . what am I mad at *you* for?"

"Because you're *insane!*" I said, then grabbed Paul's stuff and bolted for the door.

SURVIVAL TIP #30

Short of the roof caving in, the most dangerous situation you could find yourself facing in a gym would be a confrontation with a habitual steroid user. Juice-heads tend to be huge (often 250-300 lbs. or more), strong, and savage once provoked. And the buckets of testosterone and estrogen pumping through their bloodstream make it all too easy to piss them off. Worse, their responses to (real or imagined) slights are often disproportionately brutal.

I've seen bodybuilders fly into rages, lashing out at others with all their strength, just because they were teased. Believe me, getting sucker punched by a 300 lb. weightlifter who can bench 500+ is no joke. Even a slap from such a behemoth is enough to break a man's jaw. You want to avoid playing "David" to your gym's resident "Goliath."

Choose your words carefully, because juiceheads have wildly fluctuating hormone levels that make them hypersensitive. If you joke around and they misinterpret you, they're bound to overreact.

Trust me, you won't be laughing when your jaw is wired shut.

RECREATIONAL DRUG USE

All sorts of recreational drugs make their way into gyms for people to use – often by the employees.

I worked very briefly with a young saleswoman at Empirical Sports. When I say briefly, that's because her employment lasted only three days.

"Barbie" was a pretty blonde with large breasts. When my manager hired her, he informed me that, despite the tremendous pressure our salespeople were under, he was sure she'd last and do great. With her looks, physique, and winsome smile, she was a natural. What he *didn't* know, however, was that Barbie was a cocaine cowgirl and that, when subjected to a lot of stress, she'd seek out her favorite remedy.

One day, after being castigated for not hitting the numbers, Barbie came staggering out of the ladies room with some powdery substance coating her nose, lips and chin.

And it *wasn't* chalk.

She plopped down in her office chair, swaying back and forth like a sapling in a stiff breeze, and started flirting with every man that passed by. Her words may have been slurred, but when she started stripping and fondling her breasts, there was little doubt what she was trying to communicate.

Unfortunately for the eager audience that had gathered, she soon dropped onto her desk like she'd been tasered and passed out.

Of course, our manager flipped out and she was fired immediately. But the rest of us took great enjoyment in rewinding the lobby security footage so we could watch her peel open her blouse and hoist up her melons, again and again.

Most of the time, though, we wouldn't catch drug users in the act. We'd just find the evidence.

One of the employees at Caveat Sports apparently had a big-time heroin problem. We found out about it after the cleaning staff discovered a collection of blood-soaked needles concealed in the drop ceiling directly above the nursery. I was speechless. The image of kids frolicking in a room with heroin-laced needles hovering just a few feet over their heads was not exactly comforting.

At Empirical Sports, I found a whole cache of drugs stashed inside the drop ceiling – marijuana, crack cocaine, and Lord knows what else. The drugs were concealed inside tampons (of all things), and there were opened cans of coffee placed all around the stash. I was told that the aroma of coffee grounds apparently conceals the smell of the drugs, preventing people walking around the gym floor from realizing that ten grand of crank and cannabis was sitting on top of their heads.

Some people will stop at nothing to spice up their workout.

Over the years I caught plenty of people in the act of snorting, ingesting and injecting all sorts of goodies – usually in closets and bathroom stalls. My absolute favorite story has nothing to do with *using* drugs, though. It's about a person who was more of what you'd call a distributor.

And a ballsy little entrepreneur she was.

ABSOLUTELY PRICELESS: THE DEALER

A few chapters ago, I mentioned a receptionist at Empirical Sports named "Sunny." I always enjoyed working with this hellion. She was a riot – outspoken, brazen, and had a mouth that would make a pimp blush. She was equally popular with the rest of my staff. One of the front desk associates – a cantankerous, older gentleman named "Cassidy" – used to leave her love notes. One day, I found a message he'd taken for her. It read: "*Sunny, your dentist called, you bitch.*" I saved that note for years, and pulled it out of my desk whenever I needed a good laugh.

Sunny was also ambitious – and evidently unsatisfied with her mini-mum-wage Empirical Sports salary. She decided to start "supplementing" her income.

As I was leaving work one "sunny" afternoon, I noticed something in the parking lot.

Sitting in a chair there, with her back to the fence, was Sunny. That was the first thing that struck me as strange – she'd brought an office chair out-side. Stranger still was the line of men standing before her. At the head of the line, directly in front of Sunny, a guy was "posing" with his feet shoulder width apart and his arms folded across his chest.

And Sunny had her head down.

I felt a spike of panic. From the guy's pose and Sunny's positioning, it looked like she was going down on him. I started walking toward them, all the while praying, *"Oh God, please don't let this girl be giving assembly-line blowjobs in my parking lot!"*

I drew closer, dreading what awaited me. The guys spotted me and scattered like roaches. Sunny, oblivious, continued on about her business. As I got closer I saw what she was doing. She wasn't turning tricks – in-stead, she had a huge bag of marijuana and some rolling papers piled up in her lap.

The lunatic was rolling joints and selling them right there in the parking lot, in broad daylight! Plus, I recognized that one of the guys in line was a cop!

With my jaw hanging, I walked up to her. She was so busy licking and sealing that fat doobie I could have done the Macarena naked and she'd have just kept going. She kept her head down, extended one hand out in warning, and muttered gruffly, "Back off. Don't *crowd* me."

At this point my temper got the better of me. I sucked in a huge breath and bellowed, "What the *fuck* are you doing?"

Marijuana flew in every direction as Sunny screamed and heaved back in her chair, eyes wide and clutching her heart. It took her a few seconds to realize she hadn't been busted, and she sputtered, "Holy fucking shit – thank God it's only you!"

"Yeah . . . thank *God*," I said. "Now clean up your traveling sideshow and get out of here before you get us both in trouble."

For the record, I didn't call the police or rat her out. It just wasn't my style.

Of course, that doesn't mean I let that sociopath continue running her little pharmacy on club property.

I do have *some* principles.

CHAPTER 21:

CANCELING YOUR MEMBERSHIP

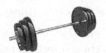

All things eventually yield to the ravages of time, be it a star in the heavens or a gym membership. Say you want to cancel your health club contract – perhaps due to dissatisfaction, time constraints, a bad breakup, or maybe even something you learned from the pages of this book.

Can you do so? And what will happen?

Over the course of this chapter we'll take a look at cancelations in detail, including what to watch for when canceling and some tried and true techniques to keep you out of trouble along the way.

PHONE CANCELS = PHONEY CANCELS

We know that health clubs make most of their money from their client's gym dues. That being the case, you can bet your gym shorts they're going to make it hard for you to cancel. Expect to jump through a frustrating series of hoops.

The first hoop will be their customer service line. If you're a member of a larger chain and want to rid yourself of your contract, calling their 800 number might seem like the best route.

It's not.

Most health club memberships can only be canceled via registered or certified mail, not over the phone. It's spelled out in your contract. Think about it – if people could call up and cancel whenever they felt like it, every gym in the country would have to close their doors.

If you do call, the odds of talking to a human being are slim. Most of the larger chains have plenty of defenses set up to deter you from quitting. When you dial in you'll be put on hold by an automated system. You'll hear a long, mealy-mouthed message from the company, touting their dedication to your health and well-being, followed by elevator music. Finally, as frustration claws at your resolve, you'll push buttons in the desperate hope it will finally transfer you to the desired department.

Then you'll be put on hold again – and usually for a long time.

When I worked at Empirical Sports, infuriated members often told me they'd waited for someone to pick up for twenty minutes or more. After all of that, many had somehow been "disconnected" and had to call back again. I believe them, because the same thing often happened to *me*. In my opinion, this is done deliberately to wear clients down and discourage them from getting the information they need. As I said, you can't cancel over the phone. But the owners don't want you to know that. They want you to just keep calling until you give up.

And it often works.

It's a matter of pain vs. pleasure. Time is precious – and you just wasted thirty minutes. With more important things to do, you throw up your hands and tell yourself you'll try again tomorrow. But tomorrow turns into a month, maybe even two or three. And all the while you're still paying dues.

Anyone you get on the line will undoubtedly be slippery. After they try to discover the real reason you're quitting, they'll throw enticements at you to convince you to stay. This may include free personal training sessions, a discounted monthly rate (locking you in for at least another year), freezing your contract, or other tricks.

A word to the wise: If you get through on the phone, do *not* fall for it if customer service tells you they'll cancel your membership by phone – there's a 99% chance that they're either lying or an idiot. After all, their job is to keep you from canceling. If you're promised a phone cancelation, be smart and get it in writing, either via email or fax. You'll want proof, because when the company tries to stick it to you later, you'll have some serious ammo to use against them.

Some people call the local club instead of the customer service line. They wager that since it's where they spend their money, they'll be treated better.

It's a lousy bet.

Things will turn out equally bad. The receptionist will tell you that only the manager is allowed to do cancelations. And the manager will *never* be at his desk. You can leave messages every day for a year – he won't call you back. Think about it: you could cost him his bonus, so why should he help you?

To be sure, there are ways around this. I advised clients to mislead the receptionist into believing that they were interested in joining. They'd call back and tell her, "I'd like to talk to the manager about a membership." Predictably, my boss would hop on that phone faster than a fat kid on a Twinkie. The best part of this gambit was that technically my client wasn't lying.

They *were* calling about a membership – theirs.

Of course, my manager wasn't happy about it. But at least my client had him in their sights.

TYPES OF CANCELATIONS

Make sure you follow your club's specific rules and regulations in order to get the job done.

Let's look at your two basic options:

- Non-commit cancels. These are either for pay-as-you-go memberships (not sold by all companies), or term contracts that have passed their initial date of obligation. A good example of the latter is a standardized one-year commit which converts to non-commit status after twelve months.
- Commit cancels. These are committed memberships that are still under contractual obligation. The term might range anywhere from twelve months (the norm) to thirty-six (a Caveat Sports staple).

  You typically perform non-commit cancels by sending a letter stating your wish to cancel via registered or certified mail. Some companies also allow their members the option to cancel in person.

Editor's Note: This gives them the chance to talk you out of canceling face to face.

If done in writing, the notice of cancelation must usually be sent to the company's corporate office, along with the original copy of the contract (save a photocopy for your records), your membership card, and payment of any owed dues. Again, make *sure* you send it certified.

Using certified mail serves dual purposes. Besides being a requirement, per your contract, it lets you know your cancelation request got there. It also gives you legal proof in case the company claims they never got it. They'll have to backdate your cancelation to the date it originally arrived.

Having a copy of your contract is especially important. Besides the fact that most chains request its return when you cancel, it also gives you the address of their corporate office and spells out any additional terms that may be required to cancel (This is why many gyms like to avoid giving you your paperwork – it makes it that much harder for you to leave).

Typical terms of cancelation are thirty days from receipt of notice, although I've seen them run sixty or even more. Be mentally prepared to shell out for another month or more once you do decide to quit.

Commit cancels are far trickier. Usually, the only ways to get out of these are via medical reasons or moving (or at least pretending to move) outside the range of their clubs.

Be careful. If the club owners own another chain within range of your new address, technically you could be forced to keep your membership. Many of the larger chains have so many locations you'd have to move to the wilds of Montana to escape them.

Typically you have to move your permanent residence at least twenty-five miles from any club owned or operated by the seller. Otherwise, they'll keep on billing you, which can really suck. Think about it: if there's a club *twenty-four miles* from you, you'll have to either drive there every day or eat the loss. I know of a former gym owner who closed down two of his clubs after pushing "discounted" early-bird renewals for six months straight. The only club he kept open was within twenty-five miles of the others.

Quite cunning.

That way he could shut down or sell off his less profitable locations, while keeping everyone's money. And it was perfectly legal! There was nothing anyone could do about it. Once all the contracts had expired, he shut down his final club and vanished. People showed up and found padlocks on the door and all the equipment gone.

And it *all* happened in the middle of the night.

To cancel for relocation you have to provide proof – a copy of a driver's license, utility bill, lease, or mortgage. If you *already* live far away (or have an out-of-state driver's license), be smart and keep that info to yourself; otherwise it can come back to bite you. I've seen managers tell people, "I'm really sorry, but *technically* you're not relocating. You already lived at this address when you joined . . ."

My clients at Empirical Sports loved me because I was on their side. Once I found out someone was in town from, say, Miami for five months, I'd tell them right away to use their girlfriend's New York address and keep that Florida driver's license well hidden. It would come in handy when they were ready to cancel.

The other way to cancel a commit membership is for medical reasons. Typically, you must be unable to use the club's services for a period of at least six months. Proof of disability is required – this means a doctor's note.

Some demanding contracts require "significant physical disability" to cancel, like at Caveat Sports. An old girlfriend of mine had an accident at one of their Manhattan locations. A leg machine had a pin jammed in its weight stack and no one was there to help her. When she tried to wrestle it out herself some plates fell on her wrist, nearly breaking it. She tried to cancel because she was hurt, but the company refused – even though her doctor stated she couldn't work out. Caveat Sports' corporate office wrote back that she was still able to use the "majority of their services": the sauna, the showers, and the leg machines. Therefore she was still obligated to stay. It wasn't until I wrote a letter for her, hinting at a potential lawsuit, that they finally let her out of her contract.

After that, I made it a point to always help clients who needed to cancel for medical reasons. If their note was insufficient, I'd steer them in the right direction. For example, I'd have their doctor write down that they were "unable to exercise until further notice" – it sounds much more severe and professional.

Don't you think?

SURVIVAL TIP #31

Some people, unable to cancel their contract, simply decide to stop paying. If they're being billed via EFT, this can be hard. Billing departments are usually very aggressive when it comes to getting clients' money – even if it means manually resubmitting your dues to your credit card (charging you an extra fee for doing so). I was once erroneously billed for a friend's membership for a year straight. I finally had to cancel the credit card in order to stop the charges – and even then they kept trying to bill me. Eventually, my card company sent them a nasty letter, ordering them to cease and desist.

If you do manage to stop paying without formally canceling, you're not out of the woods yet. Most health club chains use collection agencies that will gladly haunt you until the day you die. When I left Caveat Sports, I bought a cheap membership so I could keep training until I got my next job. Since I knew I'd renege on my contract, I used a non-existent phone number, gave no billing info, and even signed with my non-dominant hand. Seven years later, they were still sending me threatening notices. And not just to me – to my father's and brother's houses as well.

On slow days, I used to call this collection agency and taunt them. Foaming at the mouth, they demanded my phone number (so they could threaten me directly instead of through nasty letters). I'd chuckle and say, "What's that? You'd like my home number? Sure, why not? Hey, while we're at it, would you like my credit card number and banking info – maybe the keys to my car, too?"

As luck would have it, that defaulted membership did stay on my credit report for a full seven years. But back then my credit score was so abominable I didn't really care.

To get out of a binding agreement, it's better to either "move" to your friend's place in Timbuktu (having him put one of his utility bills under your name works nicely) or find a friendly doctor and go the medical route (cough, cough!). It might require a little effort, but it'll save you a lot of grief in the long run.

ABSOLUTELY PRICELESS: THE MOTHER OF ALL CANCELS

The worst cancelation horror story came from a client of mine.

Let's call her "Andy."

One day, Andy walked into my office at Empirical Sports and expressed an interest in signing up. I could see right away that she was a little gun-shy, so I tried to make her comfortable. Eventually, she relaxed enough to ask me if I recognized her. When I said "no," she explained why she was hesitant about joining. It turned out she'd been on a local investigative news program, which was similar to *Help Me Howard*.

Amusingly, she ended up on the show because of my old buddies at Caveat Sports. She'd gone to one of their clubs as a paying guest, but lost interest after seeing the place. As she put it, it was "smelly, gross and disgusting, and the people were obnoxious and rude." She left the club minus her twenty-dollar guest fee and happily went on with her life.

Three months later, Andy received threatening notices in the mail from "Borderline Credit," Caveat Sports' pet collection agency. They claimed she owed close to two thousand dollars from her gym membership, calling her house, her parents' place, her job . . . you name it.

Confused, Andy contacted Caveat Sports directly, only to be told she'd purchased a three-year contract and then reneged on her agreement. They said it was already on her credit report and threatened to sue if she didn't pay. After some investigating, she found out that the sales rep she spoke to three months earlier had signed her up without her knowledge or consent. He took the personal info she'd given him on her guest card, used her guest fee as the down payment, and forged her signature on the contract. All so he could get his pathetic little commission.

Andy requested and received a copy of "her" contract, and easily proved that the signature wasn't hers. Caveat Sports' corporate office didn't care. They insisted she owed them the money – if she didn't pay they would destroy her credit and take her to court.

Andy told me that the next three months were like beating her head against a stone wall. Finally, out of desperation, she went to the media. The news crew did an investigation and then went to the club that victimized her, shoving their cameras in the manager's face. With public opinion turning against them, someone from Caveat Sports' corporate office made an appearance on the news, claiming that the "poor girl" had been victimized by a "disreputable salesperson" who'd been righteously fired. The corporate suit claimed they would do everything in their power to undo the harm, including on her credit report.

Maybe that guy should run for President.

Editor's Note: Be extremely careful about what personal information you give to a health club – especially one you're just visiting. And be even more so if you've heard bad things about the place.

Trust your judgment. Your instincts are probably right. Gyms are like loose men and women. They don't have tawdry reputations for no good reason.

They earn them.

CHAPTER 22:

MY FINEST MOMENTS

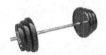

When I talk about my long and arduous career in fitness, most people scoff or even call me a bald-faced liar. They say, "Things like that just don't happen in real life – even in health clubs. Or, if they do, it's only on cheesy reality TV shows."

Unfortunately, they're mistaken.

Here are a few of my career "highlights" I'd like to share with you. Some of them made me laugh so hard I pretty much pissed myself. And others were so outright insane they emotionally scarred me for life.

Enjoy.

CHARACTER SPOTLIGHT: THE BEAST FROM THE EAST

Health clubs gather an incredibly diverse collection of individuals under one roof. People congregate there who under normal circumstances would never associate with one another. Race, religion, politics, and even economic status are no barriers. You'll see doctors, mechanics, actors, priests, police officers and drug dealers, all working out side by side.

With a few lunatics thrown in.

One client who used to scare the *hell* out of me was an oversized Asian woman named "Beijing Betty." Betty was infamous for terrorizing the halls of Empirical Sports. It wasn't because of her physique (the woman weighed 220 and was built like a sumo wrestler). It was because Betty was *psychotic*. In my humble opinion, she'd crossed the border from reality to insanity years ago – and decided she liked where she was.

Betty was trouble from day one, when she approached my new front desk girl in the locker room and gave her a big girl-on-girl hug to welcome her aboard.

Mind you, they were both buck-naked at the time.

Horrified, the poor receptionist told me about Betty's thick mess of stringy pubic hair – an eight-inch black curtain dense enough to twirl your fingers around (not that she wanted to). That in addition to her smelling like a garlic-and-rotten-fish stew.

A few weeks later, Betty revealed her disturbing habit of walking out of the ladies locker room onto the gym floor during rush hour.

Naked as a jay bird, of course.

Editor's Note: Why is it things like this never involve a smoking-hot Japanese girl in need of directions?

Betty's au naturel appearance inspired sheer panic. My first instinct was to grab a high-powered tranquilizer gun, dart her from a safe distance, and then tag her ear. But as this behemoth lumbered toward me, her shuddering folds of gelatinous genital fat completely exposed, my courage evaporated like drops of sweat hitting hot asphalt. The members had to put on imaginary blinders and trained as if their very lives depended on it.

Which they may very well have.

Fortunately for all of us, female staff members were close at hand each time this nightmare unfolded. They had the presence of mind to throw an arm over Betty's broad shoulders and rush her back into the locker room.

My own problems with Betty started a few months later. After I tried to sign her up for PT, she developed a bizarre crush on me. I recognized this immediately and, in the interest of self-preservation, fled the gym whenever she showed up. One day, however, she caught me off guard and cornered me in my office. She told me she had a "business proposition" for the company and wanted to run it by me.

As I sat there, trying to be diplomatic and breathing through my mouth, Betty pitched me her plan. Apparently, she'd recently watched a series of documentaries on the Vietnam War and was touched by the plight of the "poor Viet Cong" as they fought against the "disgusting, evil Americans" using "bamboo sticks against jet fighters." She wanted to do something to help the Vietnamese children who'd suffered during the war; namely, take them to Disneyland, with my company footing the bill. After that, she planned on expanding her "organization." She also intimated that she didn't want to do the actual *work* of promoting her impromptu charity; she just wanted was to be the "pretty face" on its posters and ads.

As I stared into Betty's beady eyes, I couldn't decide whether to chuckle or vomit. Although her anti-American comments rankled me, the notion of my bosses shelling out money for her ridiculous fantasy was comical. It was the "pretty face" bit, however, that really set my jaw aching from biting down so hard – the only way I could keep from laughing in her face.

I leaned forward and formed a steeple with my fingers. "Hmm. Well, Betty, I'm a little . . . confused. If you and the Vietnamese hate America so much, why would you want to take them to Disney? It's an American institution."

She dismissed that fact and said she'd take them to Disney in China or Japan instead – *they* would accept the poor Viet Cong children with open arms. I nodded.

"Well, Betty, that's very nice," I said. "But didn't the war in Vietnam end some forty years ago?" Before she could respond, I slammed the lid shut on her and grabbed my nail gun. "So, these "*poor children*" you're referring to are basically middle-aged adults, now – assuming they're still alive. Tell me something: do you even *know* what year it is?"

Betty recoiled in her seat, nearly shattering my poor office chair. From her expression, I could tell that she would explode at me if I gave her a moment to recover. Instead, I let her have it with both barrels.

"Listen, lady . . . I don't care what twisted fantasies you choose to live out in that warped mind of yours, but I'm not about to listen to any more of your anti-American rhetoric. So take your big, hate-filled ass and get the *hell* out of my office!"

Betty didn't say a word. She studied me intently, and then got up and left. I hoped that would be the end of it, but I had made a serious miscalculation. Everyone else was scared of her – especially once they realized she was a few beers short of a six-pack. But because I stood up to her, she became fixated on me. Her crush turned into an *obsession*. She stalked and harassed me for the next six months, leaving perverse messages for me with the receptionist, and calling me from blocked numbers while she masturbated.

The best Betty story took place eighteen months later. She'd long since disappeared from the gym, and the bizarre sex calls had vanished.

Unaware of what was to come, I was down on one knee behind the front desk, preparing to slide an envelope of cash into the club safe. Above me stood two of my co-workers, a personal trainer named "Mark," and a front desk associate named "Flip." As I completed the drop, I heard an unmistakable bellow as Betty stomped up the steps of my club.

"Where the fuck is Max?" she roared. "I got a *bone* to pick with him!"

A vision of Betty picking her teeth with my ribs flashed through my head. "Oh shit!" I threw myself on the floor, praying that the front desk and my two colleagues would keep her from spotting me.

Mark and Flip, realizing my plight, saved my ass by blocking Betty's view. As they stood shoulder to shoulder, I wiggled sideways like a frightened worm and worked my way behind the desk, pressing myself tightly against its dusty laminate.

Betty roared, and as images of the T-Rex attack from "Jurassic Park" swam before my eyes, I squeezed my 200 lb. frame under the front desk.

Editor's Note: This is a grown man so afraid of a woman he'd lay on a dirty floor for ten minutes and cram his body into a ball, just to avoid a confrontation.

As I cowered there, things above me quickly went from bad to worse. After seeing my office was empty, Betty turned on the two guys shielding me – Mark in particular. A vicious argument broke out within seconds. Mark was African American, and I could hear her getting "street" with him. She said, "Listen, *bro*, you don't know who you messing with. Don't make me have to get all ghetto and bust a cap in your black ass, 'cause you won't know what fucking hit you! You got me?"

I could tell that Mark, a formerly convicted felon, was getting nervous. This was understandable; he was dealing with a lunatic after all. To his credit, he protected me, while I hid like a frightened squirrel. As things intensified, I remember shaking my head and thinking, "My God, is a race riot brewing right over my head?"

Thankfully, the front desk guy stepped in and played peacemaker. A minute later, Betty espied our new Hispanic sales rep, and her fury faded as she invaded his office. She was a fickle creature, and her "love" for me vanished at the sight of her new Don Juan. Taking advantage of this distraction, I sprint-crawled into the nursery to hide with the rest of the frightened children.

Thank God Betty didn't notice me – the nursery had no back door. She'd have had me cornered, and I'd have worn out my teeth chewing an exit through the drywall.

THROWN UNDER THE BUS

In the fitness industry, two things are most likely to put your job at risk. The first is failing to perform as required, especially in sales or management. The second is the stupid shit that comes out of your mouth.

At one point I worked with a female sales rep named "Fannie." Fannie was a fun-loving girl with a reputation for several things: her bodacious breasts, her self-professed taste for well-hung men, and her utter lack of bootie.

It was a running joke among the staff that, although Fannie was attractive, she had no ass whatsoever. And I am *so* not kidding. When the mood struck her she'd sit in my lap – and the bones down there absolutely *killed* me. I thought I was being stabbed. My manager Sal and his assistant "Mack" joked that she suffered from an "ass deficit" and that she owed the bank ass, like a defaulted loan. When the bills came in, we'd crack up and pretend they were for all the ass she owed.

On one of my days off, Fannie was hanging out in Sal's office. He started ribbing her about – of all things – her butt. Being Fannie, she decided to give him a dose of his own medicine. She gave Sal an earful about his tiny penis. Although she'd never seen it, she said she could tell – women have a sixth sense about such things, and she *knew* he was hung like a field mouse.

She must have struck a nerve. Unwilling to let Fannie one-up him, Sal retaliated, unfortunately sacrificing me and Mack in the process.

"Oh *yeah?*" Sal sniggered. "Well, *you* should know that yesterday Mack was in here, rubbing that big delivery box behind you. And *he* said it felt just like your *butt*. And three weeks ago, *Max* said you have the ass of a twelve-year-old *boy!*"

How do I know he said this? First thing in the morning that following Monday, my office door burst open as if a SWAT team was coming through. It was Fannie, wearing a look that promised absolute death and destruction.

"*ASS like a twelve-year-old BOY?*" she snarled.

My eyes popped out of my head. Although I tried to appear calm, I found myself thinking: *"Unemployment line, here we come!"*

Fannie laid into me, pure outraged womanhood as she recounted what had gone down between her and Sal. At first I said nothing. I just sat there, rigidly upright, thinking, *"Fucking Sal ... just wait until I get my hands on him, that backstabbing piece of shit ..."*

I mean, *really?* What kind of a world is it that we live in when a couple of guys can't make fun of a chick behind her back without someone running to her like a gossipy washwoman?

Naturally, I had little time to dwell on such things – I was in full survival mode. No longer frozen like a "deer in the headlights," I did what any red-blooded American male would do in my place: deny, deny, *deny*.

As soon as Fannie realized that a signed confession wasn't forthcoming, she changed tactics. She tearfully told me that she'd "always looked up to me as a big brother," and that "it was very hurtful that I'd said such things."

Eventually, after she finally calmed down, I discovered that Fannie was so irate because she had a serious crush on me (hence the whole lap-sitting thing). And once she found out that I wasn't interested in her sexually, she understandably got upset.

I may be cheap, but I'm not easy.

A BITCH NAMED KARMA

Sometimes it seems God has a particularly wicked sense of humor. And occasionally you find out that you don't have to say a word to end up with your ass in a sling.

Pantomiming will do just fine.

One day, I was relaxing in my office, chewing the fat with Lance, an Empirical Sports sales colleague. You may remember Lance from one of our previous chapters; he's the one who used to drag his female colleagues into storage closets so he could ravage them.

As we remarked on the girls walking by, Lance spotted a very pretty brunette going towards the exit. "Oh God, I would *love* to take a big bite out of her ass," he said.

To accentuate this, Lance pushed himself up out of his chair using just his arms – like he was doing a dip – and ecstatically "chomped" in her direction. Suddenly, his face became panic-stricken and turned a brilliant scarlet.

"Omigod, she saw me!" he stammered.

As I followed his line of sight, I realized our fine lady had been covertly watching Lance in the reflection of the glass doors. She'd seen his antics in full detail.

Of course, I laughed uproariously.

The girl never turned back; she just kept walking. But poor Lance was ready to crawl into a hole and die. He spent the next few days dreading whether she would call our manager or corporate to complain.

Fortunately, neither of these things came to pass.

As divine providence would have it, I was punished myself soon thereafter. The very next day, I was in *his* office when the most amazing girl walked by. This babe had a rump you could rest a beer on, a rack that put Pamela Anderson's to shame.

I was so enthralled I couldn't help myself.

As soon as "Pamela" passed us, I went on and on about her, confessing how I longed to gently bring her to her knees, make love to her glorious face, and hose down her magnificent bombs with hot pints of man-goo. To better illustrate my point, I acted out my desires, stroking my imaginary member with gusto.   Unbeknownst to me, my heart's desire had spun around and seen my entire performance from a front row seat. Our eyes met through the glass of Lance's office, and I felt my stomach drop. I didn't know *what* to do. I was frozen in fear, hand hovering over crotch, as I waited for her to raise hell.

Fortunately, the chick burst out laughing, gave me a huge smile, and then continued on her way. I collapsed into the nearest chair, resting my hand over my heart and praying my blood pressure would return from the ionosphere. In the end, we both were saved by the same thing. Both our girls had wild and rowdy senses of humor and thought the attentions they were getting were hilarious.

I guess it didn't hurt that we were both tall, cute, and built. Otherwise, things might have been a little less pleasant.

ABSOLUTELY PRICELESS: MY BALL'S IN YOUR COURT

One of the most insane things I've ever witnessed *anywhere* took place on the racquetball courts at Dinar Fitness.

It was busy, the club was bustling, and everyone was in a good mood. I had no clients at the time, so I popped down to the gym floor to stretch my legs and see what was cooking.

As I passed the racquetball courts, I noticed three guys playing triplets. They were regulars: stocky senior citizens with thin hair and fat wallets. I gave them a glance – then came to a screeching halt. I did a double take, rubbing my eyes to make sure I wasn't seeing things.

All three of them were nude.

With the exception of their court shoes (traction is important) and racquets, they were naked as jaybirds. I looked wildly about to see who would stop them, but nothing was being done. In fact, eight people were sitting there watching the game, smiling and laughing like everything was completely normal.

Even stranger, the rest of the gym didn't seem to notice, either.

I thought I'd lost my mind. Had reality just flown out the window? The oldsters kept serving (imagine if one of them caught the return low?) and volleying back and forth in their white-walled nudist colony. And outside, members walked by like it was no big deal. Male or female, they'd stroll to the water fountain, glance at the court, and then walk on as if it were the most natural thing in the world.

I couldn't understand it (Maybe if the guys had been lean, muscular athletes, instead of paunchy, winkled up has-beens, the women would have been more interested).

Appalled and bewildered, I rushed upstairs and told my manager. He shook his head and chuckled. "Yeah, they do that periodically. The guys on the court lost a bet with the rest of their league, and now they gotta pay up!"

After hiding out for twenty minutes, I chanced an uneasy glance onto the court below – the three geriatrics were still going at it. And let me tell you, all that shifting about as they lunged for shots was a sight *no* one should see. Three hot babes playing I could watch all day . . . but *this*?

To put it succinctly, there were a lot more balls than usual on the court that day . . .

From that point forward, I made it my mission to find out whatever day the racquetball league finals ended and make damn sure that I was *in absentia*. Believe me, there was *never* a better time to schedule a sick day.

OVERSIZE LOAD

Working in the fitness industry can be monotonous, so you have to come up with fun ways to break up the day – or at least to crack up your coworkers until they pee in their pants.

My office was sandwiched between two others, and had small windows that – if I got up and moved – enabled me to peek in on my coworkers. Sitting behind my desk, however, I couldn't see either of them. This was one of the company's ways to make sure their sales reps weren't sitting around and making faces at one another all day.

When the mood struck me, I'd get up and check the other offices to see who was there. Once I ascertained it was safe, I'd knock on the glass to make sure I had their attention. Then, I'd pull back out of sight and grab my trusty pump bottle of hand sanitizer. With my free hand, I'd begin softy banging against the drywall adjacent to the window. It was a light, rhythmic drumming, which I quickly accelerated in terms of both speed and intensity. When my banging got so loud that it was deafening on the other side, I'd stop and spurt three or four big pumps of sanitizer gel onto the window, allowing it to land in long arcs that dripped filthily down the glass.

The occupants of the adjoining office would instantly laugh and scream in collective horror and/or delight. I assume I don't have to explain the illusion . . .

After doing this, I'd return to the window and grin at my colleagues while pretending to adjust my pants. I'd even pretend to lick the sanitizer off the window (it was alcohol-based, and when wiped with a paper towel vanished completely, destroying any evidence).

I was invincible back then.

PIÈCE DE RÉSISTANCE

Ironically enough, my absolute, all-time favorite health club experience – one I consider to be my crowning achievement – revolved around (of all things) gym dues.

I was working at Empirical Sports at the time, a few weeks after they'd instituted their ever-popular annual dues increase (raising all their members' monthly dues by three dollars). There'd been the usual grumblings amongst our clientele, and a few calls from people who wanted to cancel because of the price hike, but nothing of any real significance.

That all changed in a heartbeat.

I was sitting in my office, sneaking in work on some outside project, when a muscle-headed cujine wearing a white "wife-beater tank-top" suddenly burst in on me.

"We got a fucking problem!""Cujine" bellowed, looming angrily over me.

"I beg your pardon?" I asked. Had I unknowingly slept with his wife or girlfriend?

"*You*," Cujine continued, pointing a stubby finger at my nose. "You raised my fucking dues!"

"I did *what?*"

"You heard me. You raised my dues . . . tree bucks a month!"

I breathed a sigh of relief. At least I understood the source of the guy's ire now – even though it was totally misdirected.

I shifted in my seat. "Sir, I had nothing to do with raising your dues. The company-"

"Bullshit, you raised my fucking dues!"

"The *company* raised your dues," I repeated irately. "It's completely beyond my control. In fact, if you look at your contract, it-"

"I don't give a *shit* what my contract says," Cujine growled. "I'm holding *you* responsible."

I felt my aggravation building. It had been a great day up until now, but the sheer stupidity of this guy was starting to grate on my nerves.

"Is that right?" I asked. My eyes narrowed. "And what do you suggest we do about that?"

"*You're* gonna lower my dues," Cujine announced smugly. He obviously figured his steroidal physique and audacious tirade had managed to intimidate me.

He couldn't have been more wrong.

"Oh *am* I?" I replied with a little smile. "And *how* do you suggest we do that?"

"I dunno," Cujine said, shifting his weight back and forth. "But I ain't leaving this office until we figure outta way that you're gonna lower my dues."

"Oh, really?" I leaned contemplatively back in my chair.

"Really."

Out of nowhere, an absolutely evil thought sprang into my head. It was an awful (albeit tantalizing) idea, one rife with disaster, and almost certain to cost me my job if I succumbed to the temptation.

So, naturally, I succumbed.

"Okay . . ." I drawled. Remaining seated, I gently kicked out with my feet, sliding my chair a few feet to the right, and leaving my entire lower body exposed.

Without another word, I reached down and yanked open my zipper. Then I sat there with my hands resting on my thighs and an expectant, "come hither" look on my face.

There were a few seconds of silence as I looked my Neanderthal nemesis in the eye and gave him an inviting smirk. I figured there was a 70% chance he'd come charging at me like a bull. I waited for it, and planned on stopping him with a hard straight right to the jaw, followed by bouncing his head off the edge of my desk until he lost consciousness.

Cujine turned beet red and swelled up like an angry bullfrog. His eyes widened, bulging out of their sockets in ill-contained fury. But then, instead of rushing me like I expected, he wheeled around and stormed out of my office.

"I guess *not!*" I yelled after him.

Wouldn't you know it, I never saw him again.

And good riddance.

Come to think of it, as I calculated the odds, I never gave any thought to what I'd have done if the psychotic son of a bitch decided to drop down on his knees and take me up on my "offer."

After all, *anything* is possible in the gym . . .

CHAPTER 23:

"IT IS A FAR, FAR BETTER THING . . ."

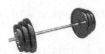

Not to toot my own horn, but looking back on my last few years in the fitness industry, I have to say I had a damn good thing going. When you consider that I'd given up on veterinary school and had a more-or-less useless degree, I was doing okay. I was making decent money, winning every award my company offered (whether I wanted them or not), and had tons of friends and hook-ups out the yin-yang.

I remember the hook-ups most fondly.

By repeatedly declining promotions and steadfastly refusing to leave my home club, I had built up an extensive network of clients, many of whom were prominent business owners. I took good care of them, and they took very good care of me. I had unparalleled connections – whatever I wanted I got. Five different restaurants sent me free food, which I lavished upon my overworked and underpaid staff. I got complimentary movie tickets and massages, free drinks at nightclubs, and huge discounts on cars, clothes, and big screen TVs.

It was like being a celebrity (except with a lot less money).

I even had a little pro bono employment agency that I used to help out my people. If a client needed a job or couldn't afford their membership, I just picked up the phone and called one of my guys. Contractors, realtors, restaurant owners . . . I had a highly diversified network. Within fifteen minutes I could get someone an interview – and they *always* got hired (take *that*, Mr. President!).

To my ever-loyal members, I was a bastion of my club. They constantly remarked that I was the only one they trusted, the only one they'd bring customers to, and the only one who lasted. Everyone else came and went like the tide. And they were right. Front desk staff, trainers, sales reps . . . it didn't matter. I was the backbone of the club, the glue that held it together.

I have to admit, after a while I bought into the whole "bastion" thing. After saying farewell to dozens of Area Managers, General Managers, and Assistant Managers – not to mention scores of fellow sales reps – I was starting to feel like the "Teflon Don." No matter how boisterous or cocky I got, no one could touch me. And I wasn't shy about saying it. Once, I even had the audacity to tell one of my more oppressive bosses, "Listen, big man: I've been through *ten* managers before you, and I outlasted them all. I'll outlast you, too."

Call it what you will: pride, hubris, or egomania – in the end, I believed what everyone told me – that Empirical Sports couldn't live without me. How could they? After all, I was the best of the best: a winning personality and a monstrous cash cow – one who never failed or faltered. I was more than just a cog in their machine; I was unique in the fitness industry. *I* was irreplaceable. What's more, after everything I'd gotten away with over the years, and everyone I'd seen come and go, I realized something else: I was invincible.

Or at least I thought I was.

THE STAGE IS SET

It was sudden, but my departure from the fitness industry really was long overdue. There's no denying it: after two decades of working in health clubs and having dealt with over a quarter of a million members, I was bone tired. Far worse, I was stuck in the mother of all ruts – in a jail from which there seemed to be no escape.

Sure, I had my fingers in a lot of pots, and the job came so easily to me I could spend most of my day staring into space – but I was also bored to death. Even with six weeks of vacation each year, my job was no longer fulfilling. It was a huge waste of talent. True, working there was convenient (my apartment was four blocks away) and the list of girls I'd known was amazing (my co-workers once tried and failed to name a country I hadn't dated a woman from), but none of that mattered anymore. I had settled down. And when all is said and done, how many more women could I have possibly slept with? How much more sex could I have had and still been able to feel something for someone?

The answer to both these questions is none. Believe it or not, even for a guy, eventually all the slamming and jamming becomes the same; in the end, all you really yearn for is a yin to your yang.

So I ended up leaving – but not by my choosing and (surprisingly) not even for something I'd said or done. I was the victim of something I saw happen to scores of people over the years: *political assassination*.

Not surprisingly, it was a group effort. When members of the Roman senate assassinated Julius Caesar back in 44 BC, his murder was also the result of a highly organized plot. Marcus Brutus couldn't do it alone; it took nearly sixty individuals working together – the only way to bring down such a politically powerful individual.

My adversaries had a far easier time. My ego notwithstanding, I was far from Julius Caesar, and it certainly didn't take sixty of them to bring me down. As my lawyer later said, there were three villains involved in the orchestration of my demise.

The first of these heavies was an Area Manager known as "Cagado."

I don't know which genius hired Cagado, but he knew absolutely nothing about fitness (in fact, someone told me he used to sell women's shoes, or some such thing). It soon became apparent he also knew nothing about running a business, period. The only thing he *was* good at was sleeping with his subordinates and firing those he disliked. Over an eighteen-month period I watched him mastermind the terminations of dozens of people.

Besides his other flaws, Cagado possessed the most egomaniacal, authoritarian management style I've ever seen. Not surprisingly, he rapidly became the most despised employee in the company. He took it personally. At one point, he whined to "Delilah," one of his General Managers, how every salesperson and manager from his other clubs "hated his guts." But it was okay, he said, "Because they'll all be gone soon."

Cagado didn't realize that Delilah detested him, too. She immediately informed my manager of his malevolent plan, as well as Human Resources. Predictably, HR made light of it, but I was alarmed – especially since me and my club were on his "hit list." I found it hard to believe someone could be so flat-out evil. After personally experiencing this phenomenon, however, I realized I was wrong.

I'd just enrolled a young lady only to have her call me two days later. She'd gotten a call from one of our other reps, who told her about a new sale that was significantly cheaper than what she paid. Naturally, I offered to credit her with the difference. It was company policy: if a member found out about a better deal within seven days of enrolling, we issued them a dues credit to cover the disparity in price. I'd implemented the policy numerous times by simply explaining the situation to whoever was Area Manager at the time. It had never been a problem. This time it was.

When I called Cagado he was less than cooperative. He told me he didn't give a "flying fuck" about company policy or doing the right thing. He flat-out refused to give the woman her credit, even though she was about to buy a $1,200 PT package. Instead, he started obsessing over which company employee had "betrayed us" by telling her about the current sale.

This bewildered me. When I pointed out that she still had time left on her money-back-guarantee and could simply cancel and rejoin at the new rate, Cagado actually told me, "She can cancel if she wants to, but I won't allow her to rejoin until *next* month, when a different promotion is in effect."

He wouldn't allow it? As if he had a choice in the matter . . .

Undeterred, I went to "Highway," our VP of sales, for help. Highway was stunned by Cagado's unmitigated arrogance. He kept saying, "That doesn't make sense. Why would he *say* something like that? That's a bad decision!"

Needless to say, he authorized giving my client the credit.

When Cagado found out, he immediately retaliated by trying to transfer me to another location. I steadfastly refused to be moved, and when he went higher up on the food chain, he was told to leave me be. He was surprised, to say the least, and grudgingly accepted that I was untouchable.

At least for the moment . . .

Still thirsty for blood, Cagado turned his sights on Antonia, my manager. He decided she was "too old to handle such a large club," and commenced a campaign to force her out. Antonia and I were tight, so he found himself facing a unified front.

After a year of open warfare – to him it must have seemed like he was beating his brains out against a granite wall – Cagado finally managed to infiltrate my club. He fired our current Assistant Manager and hand-picked her replacement.

"Leech" was the second villain that contributed to my final performance. And let me tell you, once injected into our midst, he was a real cancer cell.

Juiced up, covered with tattoos, and sporting a nasty disposition, Leech came across as a career criminal looking for his next score. From comments he made to me in private, I realized he'd been put there purely to stab Antonia in the back. I warned her, but she didn't believe me. All I could do was watch her back.

A few weeks after he started, Leech surprised even me. He walked into my office and, after some verbal foreplay, ordered me (at Cagado's behest) to cripple the club's sales. The two of them had hatched a plan to damage the company's existing sales model throughout their region. Once they'd bled the district to the point of bankruptcy, they planned on offering corporate their own "system" instead. The only thing I could figure was they'd look like heroes to their panicky superiors (whose publicly traded company was consistently losing money), and receive huge promotions for "saving the day."

I was speechless. I'd always thought Cagado was like his predecessor, Peter, and that he fired people purely out of sadistic malice. It never dawned on me that, by trying to fire Antonia and planting henchman at my club, he was laying the groundwork for a much bigger scheme. Or that his ultimate goal was to advance himself to a position of power through deceit and treachery.

He made a big mistake if he thought I'd go along with it.

Once I figured out how they planned on defrauding our shareholders, I ratted them out to Antonia. Later, after I'd left for the evening, she confronted Leech about it. He was furious, but of course he denied everything.

Two days later, Cagado showed up at my club and sent Antonia home early. Then, he and Leech pulled me into an office and got "Misellus," the third member of their little triumvirate, on speakerphone (Misellus, who worked for HR, was the company's glorified axe woman).

To my astonishment, the three of them had concocted sexual harassment charges against me and used them as an excuse to fire me. I laughed at the irony of the situation. Given the sexual excess I'd engaged in during my years in the industry, it was beyond poetic that they threw *that* at me.

Even more amusing, however, was the "source" of these allegations – the woman who had filed the complaint. Earlier that day, Cagado had pressured an Area Fitness Manager into writing him an email that accused me of saying and doing inappropriate things to her. When I read the email, I noticed that the woman didn't mention that she'd flirted with me for years, that she used to sit on my lap in Antonia's office while whispering suggestively in my ear, or that she'd asked me out the week before.

Despite this – and despite the fact that there was no real investigation or documentation – there was no way I could defend myself from the charges – at least not at the moment. So without further ado, I cleaned out my desk. The three stooges thought they had won.

As expected, Empirical Sports tried to prevent me from collecting unemployment benefits; they even had HR issue a formal statement that I'd been fired for cause (i.e. gross misconduct). Although they'd initially caught me off guard, I was not about to sit back and take their abuse. I got myself a good lawyer and took action against them. Despite their treachery, after two hearings in front of an Administrative Law Judge, all the allegations brought against me were dismissed.

I received all my benefits, retro pay included.

Survival Tip #32

This one's for all the victimized health club employees out there. Although a lot of people fired from gyms deserve it, many are let go out of pure spite. Evil managers and HR reps won't hesitate to railroad their enemies. They take advantage of their victims' ignorance of their rights and will launch attacks designed to baffle and overwhelm. They expect you to just put your head down and take it.

Don't.

The malevolent manager is trying to do two things: The first is to deny you your livelihood. They'll sleep like a baby as they relish the sweet memory of shafting someone they hate. The second is to screw you out of getting unemployment. This increases their enjoyment because they've left their victim with absolutely no way of supporting themselves. What's more, they get a pat on the back from upstairs for saving the company money.

If someone is planning your demise, fight back. Surreptitiously gather any documentation you can against them. If they sent you abusive, insulting, or threatening emails, save them. Forward them to your personal email address and save hard copies. If your boss gave you grief in front of witnesses, cultivate relationships with those people. Their testimony will come in handy.

An amusing footnote: gym bosses with an axe to grind often go after groups of people. It's guilt by association. If they kill off one viper, its friends will carry a grudge. To win the fight for good, they have to wipe out the entire nest.

By doing this, they inanely create an entire coalition of people who are all highly motivated to fight back. The falsely accused can then work together and pool their collective knowledge and experiences against a common foe.

If you're unjustly fired, don't slink away like a whipped dog. Gather evidence and witnesses and find yourself a good lawyer, especially one who specializes in Unlawful Termination. Learn your rights and let him be the enforcer. Believe me, that same jerk who smiled in your face when they fired you won't be laughing so hard when your lawyer serves them and their superiors with a fat, juicy EEOC lawsuit.

One or two years' salary may not make you rich, but it goes a long way. You'll sleep much better knowing justice was done. And best of all, your jerk of a former boss won't be winning popularity contests anytime soon.

Trust me.

THE BATTLE BEGINS

I'm nobody's whipping boy. After defeating Empirical Sports and their lawyers in the Unemployment Insurance arena, my attorney (known in private circles as "the Champ") and I launched formal SOX charges against the company.

Editor's Note: For the uninitiated, SOX stands for Sarbanes-Oxley Act. These are laws set up by the government specifically to protect whistleblowers like myself from being fired in retaliation by publicly traded companies.

My former boss, Antonia, aided me in the battle and eventually became a key witness. Shortly after I was axed, Cagado fulfilled his long-time dream of firing her. Predictably, he'd replaced her with his pawn, Leech. By doing so, he gave me a witness who was both privy to valuable information *and* eager to ensure his destruction. Antonia filed an EEOC lawsuit against Empirical Sports, forcing them to hire additional lawyers to fight multiple opponents.

As our investigation move into full swing and pressure mounted from the combined legal actions, interesting details began to come to light.

For one thing, I heard though the grapevine that my former employers had already received several lawsuits because of Cagado. He'd unjustly fired a lot of people, many of whom had filed suit. Like a fat bear surrounded by angry wolves, the company was desperately trying to settle these actions as fast as possible. I also found out that Cagado was not the person he pretended to be when hired. He'd provided Empirical Sports with a very professional-looking, *well-doctored* résumé, in order to illegitimately obtain his position as Area Manager. My own research also uncovered that Leech, as expected, had an extensive criminal record. His rap sheet included multiple accounts of drug trafficking, brandishing a firearm, burglary, and kidnapping.

Kidnapping?

It's a good thing for people like Leech and Cagado that background checks usually aren't required for management positions in fitness. I wonder how members who'd left their children in the daycare would have felt if they'd known this guy was running the place . . .

ENDGAME

There's no such thing as loyalty in the fitness industry. Once Empirical Sports Clubs recognized the magnitude of our legal actions and discovered the corrupt nature of the serpents in their midst, it was time for them to start cutting their losses.

In other words, heads began to roll.

The first one to go was Leech. Based on the report I got, after being dragged into the corporate office and interrogated about his involvement in the scheme, he freaked out and quit. After he left, it came to light that he and his sales reps had been embezzling money from clients, just like some of my former co-workers had, by taking their cash and giving them guest passes instead of real memberships. I heard estimates that they were each pocketing a grand a week doing this.

The next to go was Misellus, that lovely woman from HR. I fondly remember the gleefully malicious tone in her voice when she cost me my job – she even snickered when I told her I had a child to take care of. She wasn't laughing once the tables were turned, however. I heard that when they fired her, she got down on her knees and groveled, begging to keep her job, "How can you do this to me after all the terrible things I've done for you people?" she wailed.

In the immortal words of John Donne, "Never send to know for whom the bell tolls; it tolls for thee."

They saved the best for last. Fed up with shelling out settlement after settlement to pay for Cagado's assorted misdeeds, and faced with federal SOX charges on top of it, the company had at last had enough. My beloved former Area Manager was forced to announce to his entire region via conference call that he had been asked for his resignation. Considering all the unethical things he'd done and the people he'd victimized, Cagado actually had the nerve to whine afterward about how cruel the company was to force him out, especially given his current situation.

Hey, nobody told him to knock up his girlfriend.

Interestingly enough, after Cagado left the company, it was discovered that ten thousand dollars had disappeared from the club safe. Even more interesting was the fact that he was custodian of that safe.

Severance package, anyone?

As of the date of this writing, the results of my SOX case have yet to be determined. But win, lose, or draw, whatever the outcome, I rest easy knowing that those who schemed against me were ousted before they did any real harm. Thanks largely to me and my lawyer, my company's shareholders were spared any additional setbacks.

SURVIVAL TIP #33

Some of the larger health club chains have, in the spirit of capitalism, become publicly traded companies. A nice idea, until you do your research and find that, more often than not, their stocks depreciate like a deflating hot air balloon.

I'm no financial analyst, but I believe that once the PR hype fades after the initial public offering, the chains' true growth potential and popularity (or lack thereof) becomes apparent. People want to invest in a company they believe in, and word of mouth is a powerful tool.

In the past, I did some research on several fitness chains' approval ratings, and the results surprised even me. Most of them were dismal, with negative ranges of 40-80% – and sometimes higher!

The bottom line is: health club stocks are dicey. They're not designed to withstand the test of time. So if you want to invest your hard-earned money there, get yourself a qualified financial analyst first. Otherwise, you're playing financial Russian roulette with a loaded gun.

THE HYPOCRISY OF THE INDUSTRY

When people ask me why I was unjustly fired, I often find myself getting angry.

And who wouldn't?

I gave my employers many irreplaceable years of my life. I wasn't an ideal employee, but in that industry I was as good as anyone's going to get. I was trustworthy, productive and reliable. I showed up for my shift on time, I did my job, and unlike just about everyone else, I never stole a penny from my club or my clients (and believe me, I had *many* opportunities). I cared about my people and I busted my ass, hitting ridiculous numbers and helping to keep my employers afloat while the nation's economy went down the toilet. After crunching the numbers, I realized that I was grossing them well over one *million* dollars a year.

And what thanks did I get for being so loyal and productive and profitable?

They took the word of a flimflam man and his pet crook and fired me without even listening to my side of the story. I mean, of all people to trust! Cagado was a liar, a fool, and a would-be king, who hurt others to get what he wanted. His methods were so destructive that, frankly, I wouldn't be surprised if he was a health club double agent, hired to take Empirical Sports apart from the inside. But did anyone consider this or spring to my defense? "Hey, Max has been here for a long time and nothing like this ever happened before. Maybe we should look into this?"

No.

Nobody said a word. There was no investigation – just hastily concocted emails orchestrated by the real perpetrators the morning I was fired. And mind you, that took place less than forty-eight hours after I exposed their plan to scam the company.

In the end, after protecting my employers and their shareholders, I was tossed out like yesterday's garbage. And to cover their tracks, Cagado made sure to have Leech lie to my members, telling them I'd resigned on my own and "moved on to greener pastures."

Of course, that bitch called Karma has a way of dropping in on those who deserve it. The list of people who left the company since then – willingly or not – is very long. And my former region, home to the best money-making clubs in the company, is – as of this date – now rated the absolute worst. When I run into old clients on the street, they'll run up to me, hug me, and demand to know "why I quit." I'll get an earful about how much the club "sucks" since I left, how none of their revolving-door employees care about the members, and how they refuse to bring any of their friends in to join without me being there.

I smile and nod when I hear all of this – and wonder how much of it is true. But what really cracks me up is when they ask me if I can hook them up with a better deal somehow.

Even years later, "my people" still attribute divine powers to me.

EPILOGUE: THE SUM OF ALL FEARS

Sometimes I'm asked, after working in fitness for so long, "Do you miss it?"

Not a prayer, brother.

Sure, from a horny young man's perspective, it was great. I've *forgotten* more women than most men ever know, and had a boatload of fun along the way. But I really *was* just a well-lubed cog on someone's forever-turning wheel. It wasn't until I got off their "treadmill" and had some time to breathe that I finally realized how great it was being free from that microcosmic world.

Best of all, I was able to enjoy spending time with my family and my child. You see, once I'd managed to put my man-whoring days behind me, the smartest thing I did was to settle down. I was gifted with the most beautiful and precocious toddler a man could ever hope for. And, once that oversized monkey known as Empirical Sports was off my back, I was able to enjoy countless irreplaceable moments with my child that, otherwise, I'd have undoubtedly missed out on. Sales, commissions, bonuses, promotions, endless hours . . . it's all bullshit. Being with your children and seeing them grow, *that's* the stuff that really matters.

In a way, Cagado and his cronies did me a favor.

Another question I'm often asked is, "Do you have any regrets?"

Some people expect a response like, "I wasted years of my life," or "I lost some amazing women because of my arrogance." I can appreciate where they're coming from, but I don't actually feel like that. Everyone has regrets. But if I hadn't trodden the path I had, I wouldn't have the child I have. So any "wasted" years or failed relationships were necessary and worthwhile. We're all products of our collective experiences, and I wouldn't change mine for the world.

The only regret I *do* have is that I didn't leave my company years prior, and on my own terms. I had it all planned out – and particularly looked forward to singing Johnny Paycheck's "Take This Job and Shove It" during the monthly conference call. I think it would've been a huge hit.

Oh well. I guess that's one dream that will remain unrealized. This book will have to suffice in its place.

And speaking of the book . . .

Let me be clear: *Memoirs of a Gym Rat* was many years in the making. I didn't write these pages as some kind of vendetta against my previous employers, or to stop people from joining the gym; nothing could be further from the truth. I believe exercising properly is the best thing in the world. But people need to know the gym for what it is – a business, pure and simple. And the sad fact is that, to a commission-hungry sales rep, you're just a dollar sign dressed in a tank top and sweats.

Fortunately, you're better prepared for that now. When you inspect a gym, your eyes will be open. You'll know what to watch for, and be able to tell right away if the place is suitable for your needs. And when some smirking "program director" comes slithering your way, they'll find you far from helpless. You'll see right through their sales tactics, and be well equipped to counter them. You'll join only if *you* want to join, and *if* you do, it'll be with a package that best suits your needs – not their wallet.

What's more, when it comes to navigating the pitfalls of club life, whether it's coping with a dirty locker room, dealing with apathetic employees, or deflecting the amorous advances of some horny gym rat, you'll be fortified with that most wondrous of weapons: knowledge. After all, knowledge is, indeed, power. And although the truth ain't always pretty, it's usually better to know than to not.

Last but not least, I have a message for all the health club owners and managers out there. As you're reading this and gnashing your teeth (and undoubtedly trying to figure some way to boil me in oil), I'd like to share one of my favorite quotes from former U.S. President Harry S. Truman: "I don't give them hell. I just tell the truth and they think it's hell."

You see, you may not like this book, or the revelations inside, but it is what it is: the accurate reflections of someone who suffered the well-fanned flames of fitness for two decades, and who, luckily, escaped with enough of his sanity intact to write about it.

I guess, given my nature, that makes me an honorary "Son of Perdition." Hell, I've been called far worse things.

THE END

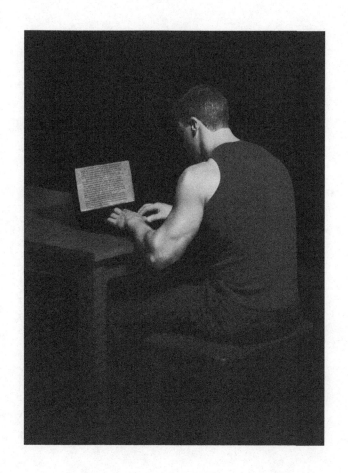

ABOUT THE AUTHOR

Max Hawthorne was born in Brooklyn, NY. He worked in the fitness industry for twenty years. He is a nationally certified personal trainer whose background includes boxing and martial arts, as well as studies in anatomy and kinesiology. In addition to penning *Memoirs of a Gym Rat,* his writing has appeared in a variety of outdoor magazines and periodicals. He is an avid sportsman and conservationist. His hobbies include hunting, fishing, and the collection of fossils and antiquities. He lives with his family in the Greater Northeast.

Made in the USA
Las Vegas, NV
02 June 2024

90623660R00164